Implementing
CLINICAL
PRACTICE
GUIDELINES

CARMI Z. MARGOLIS, MD, MA
SHAN CRETIN, PHD, MPH
EDITORS

FOREWORD BY
DONALD M. BERWICK, MD

press

Health *info*Source
An American Hospital Association Company
Chicago

© 1999 by Health *info*Source, an American Hospital Association company

Printed in the United States of America—12/98

Cover design by Amy Aves

Library of Congress Cataloging-in-Publication Data
Implementing clinical practice guidelines / Carmi Z. Margolis and Shan Cretin, editors.
p.   cm.
ISBN 1-55648-237-X
1. Medical protocols.   2. Medical care—Standards.   I. Margolis, Carmi Z., 1943–   .   II. Cretin, Shan.
[DNLM: 1. Practice Guidelines.   2. Clinical Medicine.   WB 102 I43 1998]
RC64.C549   1998
362.1'02'18—DC21
DNLM/DLC
for Library of Congress   98-19064
                                                                        CIP

Item Number: **145106**

To Adinah, an amazing choreographer, with much love
and argument

—Carmi

CONTENTS

ABOUT THE AUTHORS

Shan Cretin, PhD, MPH, is president of Shan Cretin & Associates in Santa Monica, California, resident consultant with the RAND Corporation, and an adjunct professor at the Marshall School of Business at the University of Southern California. Dr. Cretin has published numerous papers on the cost-effectiveness of preventative and curative care, quality assessment and improvement methods, and the organization and financing of care in the United States and China. She spent 15 years on the faculties of Yale University, Harvard University, and the University of California at Los Angeles. She was chair of the Department of Health Services at the University of California and co-directed the RAND/University of California Centers for Health Policy Study and Health Care Financing Research. For the past 10 years she has consulted with health care organizations in the United States and Canada, Europe, the Middle East, and Asia on methods for assessing and improving the quality of clinical care and business practices.

Carmi Z. Margolis, MD, MA, is professor of pediatrics and vice dean for medical education at Ben-Gurion University of the Negev in Beer-Sheva, Israel. While serving as founding chairman of the Division of Health in the Community, Dr. Margolis developed the clinical algorithms format later proposed as the basis for an international standard. At the same time, he embarked on cooperative research projects and visiting professorships at SUNY Downstate, University of Rochester, University of Alabama, University of North Carolina, and Harvard. At North Carolina, he was chosen as the Israel Exchange Scholar for 1982–83. He has served as chairman of the Israel Board of Pediatrics and as a consultant to the Scientific Council of the Israel Medical Association for developing primary care teaching clinics. Dr. Margolis has also been involved in developing and implementing algorithms at the Harvard Community Health Plan (now Harvard Pilgrim Health Care), at the Veterans Health Administration, and at various Israeli health plans. He is the author of *Common Pediatric*

Problems: An Algorithm Approach and *The Pediatric Problem Oriented Record,* both groundbreaking books in medical problem solving.

Robert H. Fletcher, MD, MSc, is a professor at the Harvard School of Public Health and Harvard Medical School, and also is affiliated with Harvard Pilgrim Health Care. Dr. Fletcher is a former editor of the *Annals of Internal Medicine,* the author of *Clinical Epidemiology: The Essentials,* and a co-chair of the Agency for Health Care Policy and Research Gastrointestinal Consortium for the Colorectal Cancer Screening Guideline Panel of 1997.

Carole S. Gardner, MD, is chief clinician of the Department of Practice Analysis and Support at Kaiser Permanente, Georgia, in Atlanta. Dr. Gardner, an internist and geriatrician, was on the faculty of the University of Kentucky College of Medicine before joining Kaiser Permanente. There, she served as associate director of the Department of Clinical Geriatrics at the university's Center on Aging, developing and coordinating the medical school's curriculum and its fellowship in geriatric medicine.

Donald A. Goldmann, MD, is a professor of the Department of Pediatrics at Harvard Medical School and holds the positions of medical director of the Department of Quality Improvement and vice chair of the Department of Health Outcomes, and is a member of the Department of Medicine at Children's Hospital, Boston. Dr. Goldmann has been at Children's Hospital, Boston, for the last 25 years and has served in a variety of administrative and clinical roles during this time.

Rita Gibes Grossman, RN, MSc, is a consultant at Children's Hospital, Boston. Ms. Grossman has served as director of the Clinical Practice Guidelines Program at Children's Hospital, Boston, the program coordinator for the Institute for Healthcare Improvement, analyst for the Center for Cost Effective Care and director of the Neonatal Intensive Care Unit at Brigham and Women's Hospital, a Kellogg Fellow at the Department of Health Care Policy and Management at the Harvard School of Public Health, and co-founding editor of the *Journal of Perinatal and Neonatal Nursing,* and has been a contributor of *Use of Clinical Guidelines to Promote Quality and Cost Effectiveness.*

Charles Homer, MD, MPH, is director of the Clinical Effectiveness Program at Children's Hospital, Boston, which is a part of both the Division of General Pediatrics and the Department of Hospital Epidemiology and Quality Improvement. Dr. Homer has received both federal and private funding for his studies; presently, he is principal investigator of a study funded by the Agency for Health Care Policy and Research aiming to develop and implement an automated guideline for the evaluation and treatment of hyperbilirubinemia in newborns and co-investigator of a large federally funded study aiming to develop and test measures for assessing patient preferences for health care and health plans. Dr. Homer is a consultant to the American Academy of Pediatrics in the areas of health supervision guidelines, guideline development, and functional outcome measurement. He serves as a member of the academy's Committee on Quality Improvement and chairs that committee's Subcommittee on Guideline Implementation.

Nancy Sokol, MD, is chief of internal medicine at Lahey–Concord Hillside Hospital in Concord, Massachusetts, and a member of the Board of Directors of the Lahey Clinic in Burlington, Massachusetts. She has developed and implemented clinical practice guidelines for Harvard Community Health Plan and has been on the faculty of the Institute for Healthcare Improvement as a course director for clinical quality improvement.

Dennis D. Tolsma, MPH, is director of the Department of Prevention and Practice Analysis at Kaiser Permanente, Georgia, in Atlanta. Mr. Tolsma joined Kaiser Permanente from the Centers for Disease Control and Prevention, where he held the positions of director of the Center for Health Promotion and Education and associate director for the Center for Disease Control Public Health Practice. His publications include chapters in *Public Health and Preventive Medicine* and *Environmental Medicine.*

FOREWORD

When it comes to the topic of "quality," health care can become a battlefield. Among the weapons of choice are protocols and guidelines. For many reasons, physicians especially have considered the implementation of formal care guidelines as threats—to their autonomy, to measures necessary for customizing care to the needs of individual patients, and to the "art" of medicine. The managers and other health care leaders who have attempted to introduce guidelines into care often complain that doctors are resistant or hostile to even the most basic attempts to standardize care patterns according to modern scientific guidelines.

This war, like most others, has been costly and largely unreasonable. Why should doctors, who throughout their education ask their mentors and expert advisors to offer them guidance concerning appropriate care practices, resist such guidance as that provided by formal care guidelines? Why should health care managers and clinical leaders, who employ and pay physicians to use their brains and hearts in order to continually seek better ways of caring for each patient as an important individual, worry when doctors treat guidelines as mere advice instead of as binding rules?

The tension derives not from the irrationality of doctors, managers, or guidelines themselves, but rather from the psychologic terrain of today's health care industry. The waste has been enormous. Despite millions, probably billions, of dollars spent in American health care over the past decade in order to generate guidelines of many forms and on many topics, these guidelines seem so far to have had little or no impact on care itself at most organizations in the health care industry. We find shelf after shelf full of elaborately constructed, carefully drawn, and well-documented scientific care guidelines referred to little and used less in the actual care of patients. There are exceptions, but not many.

If the use of scientific guidelines for care is sensible—and it is—and if medicine has reached a level of complexity and self-consciousness that makes carefully constructed guidelines superior in many cases to unguided individual anecdote-based opinion—and it has—then surely we can find ways to reach a truce in this war, and to act with good and common sense in order to put into practice the best aspects of the best guidelines that we can construct.

In the guidelines war, no people have more expertise in disarmament than do the authors of this book. Carmi Margolis, Shan Cretin, and their colleagues have spent nearly a decade in careful and respectful research and development of methods by which guidelines that make sense can be developed, refined, continually updated, and, most of all, put into practice in real world settings as assets in care, not as threats to the participants in care. This group of teachers and scholars has a great deal to say about the effective implementation of guidelines in the service of the improvement of health care. They have found ways, and present those ways well, for overcoming significant obstacles that have emerged through the many years of guideline warfare. Among those obstacles are the following:

1. Inefficiency abounds in methods for developing guidelines. Whereas some organizations and agencies have spent millions upon millions of dollars and several years to develop even simple guidelines, these authors offer methods by which helpful, scientifically disciplined guidelines can be written or revised within days or weeks, and thereby be much more responsive to the needs of real health care providers.
2. Whereas many guidelines enterprises have produced static rules that are unresponsive to evolving scientific knowledge, these authors offer clear approaches to the continuous tending and updating of guidelines so that they can always remain reflective of the best available knowledge.
3. Guidelines throughout the United States are developed in a panoply of inconsistent formats and styles, rendering the simple act of reading or examining a guideline for many physicians implausible. By contrast, these authors offer a clear approach to the graphical formatting and presentation of guidelines that has the capability to become an industry-wide standard. This would simplify both the production and the consumption of guidelines.
4. Many guideline developers labor mightily to author guidelines, viewing them as if they were tablets of stone sent down from a mountain of expertise to the receiving clinicians. This method works poorly, both psychologically and technically, because the very act of refinement of guidelines at a local level can often be a necessary part of adoption and adaptation. These authors describe helpful and efficient group processes, ready for use in local care settings, through which providers of care can master

and sensibly adapt guidelines to their own local needs. This process is not wasteful; it is both efficient and necessary to effective deployment.

5. Many guideline efforts are scientifically proper but "process illiterate." That is, their guideline makes sense when viewed from a pure scientific standpoint, but cannot posssibly be made real under the constraints of the work setting into which they are introduced. This is a formula for failure of implementation. These authors offer practical suggestions for assuring both the scientific pedigree and the practical usefulness of a guideline in the local care setting.

6. For the most part, efforts to introduce guidelines into practice remain underevaluated. In most settings, and for most guidelines, we have no idea whatsoever as to whether or not the intended forms of improvement of care and outcome occur as a result of offering guidelines to clinicians. These authors do not accept that degree of myopia. They insist that evaluation of effect be incorporated into efforts to introduce guidelines into real-world practices, and they offer practical advice on how the effects of guidelines can be monitored even while implementation proceeds.

This book is full of wisdom, based not upon speculation but upon experience. Its authors have helped many organizations to learn about and adapt guidelines for their own local use, and, through this book, many other organizations and health care leaders will now have the opportunity to draw much deeper and wider benefit from scientifically based care guidelines than they ever have had before.

Donald M. Berwick, MD, MPP
President and CEO, Institute for Healthcare Improvement

PREFACE

Several months ago, I asked Yitzhak Peterburg, the medical director of our university hospital in Beer-Sheva, a savvy, well-trained, and well-reputed physician administrator, whether he was interested in starting a clinical practice guideline project. He answered that he certainly was because guidelines were the wave of the future. Soon, everyone would have them. Later, at the first project team meeting, as we tried to choose a clinical topic for the first project, Yitzhak said that when you come right down to it, the reason that he needs a guideline project is to cut costs. A good project, from his point of view, would therefore be aimed at reducing use of expensive antibiotics like Fortum or reducing the length of pediatric hospitalizations. But for this first project, he hastened to add, he did not care what the topic was, as long as the project succeeded. He also mentioned that he had no intention of sponsoring the writing of new guidelines. Yitzhak felt that there were plenty of good guidelines around and that the job of a clinical guideline project director in 1996 was to tailor existing guidelines to the needs of clinicians working in a particular setting.

I reacted to my hospital director's perspective on guidelines with a pleasant sense of surprise. In our two first sessions, he had voiced basic ideas about guidelines that had taken me years to learn. He knew about choosing and designing guidelines, tailoring them, being sensitive to resistance from the medical staff, and the importance of getting them not only written but also implemented and evaluated—a far cry from what medical administrators knew about guidelines only a few years ago!

However, when I reflect on how I came to be interested in clinical practice guidelines, I realize that none of Yitzhak's correct points have played a role. For many years, I was not interested in guiding physician behavior at all. Rather, I was fascinated by the educational potential of clinical algorithms.

For me, the story begins with a routine clinical conference at Yale–New Haven Hospital's newborn nursery in 1971. As the chief resident, I listened from the back of the little conference room as the senior and the junior residents tried to decide whether to treat a newborn suffering from suspected sepsis with intravenous antibiotics. Just as they seemed to have come to an impasse, I went up to the blackboard and attempted to flow chart the argument. I explained that what they were saying was that if the baby had a statistically increased chance of sepsis, say because it had premature rupture of the membranes, then cultures should be done, but antibiotics should be withheld; however, if there was a clinical suspicion of sepsis, say because the baby was vomiting or feeding poorly or had a decreased temperature, then it should be both cultured and treated immediately.

As I completed my explanation, I heard a familiar throat-clearing and looked up to see that Dav Cook, our chief of service, had slipped into the room. "You know, Carffil, he said, "you could probably do that sort of charting for all of clinical medicine."

I spent the next 12 years learning how to construct clinical algorithms and trying to determine empirically whether they were a more effective clinical learning tool than prose or other methods for teaching how to solve clinical problems. Between 1972 and 1973, during my fellowship in medical education and cognitive psychology at Michigan State University, I continued developing what I called out of ignorance "decision trees" (and no one ever corrected me!). I succeeded in designing an experiment, later supported by the National Fund for Medical Education, that showed clinical algorithms to be both more effective and more efficient than prose for learning to solve clinical problems for which there are agreed-upon approaches to management, such as fever in a child with no other findings or bacterial meningitis.

While on sabbatical at the University of North Carolina at Chapel Hill in 1982, I often faced questions about what I was doing, and I always began my answers by spending several minutes explaining the concept of an algorithm. Four years later, in May 1986, when Steve Schoenbaum at the Harvard Community Health Plan sponsored the first of 13 workshops aimed at teaching clinicians to design and construct their own clinical algorithms, the term "clinical algorithms" was still not a familiar one. But the attitude toward them had changed. Suddenly, a large health maintenance organization was interested in them, not primarily for their applicability as teaching tools, but because they were somehow related to clinical guidelines and had the potential of reducing the extreme variations in clinical practice first demonstrated by J. E. Wennberg and A. Gittelsohn, practitioner/epidemiologists who have since mapped these variations for many common clinical problems.[1]

At the same time, the microcomputers I had first encountered at Chapel Hill were now in increasingly common use, and clinical algorithms seemed to offer a method for computerizing the clinical part of the patient record. My interest began to shift to the question of how clinicians used the algorithms they learned. Don Berwick, president and chief executive officer of the Institute for Healthcare Improvement and one of the leading figures to bring quality improvement to health care, taught me that quality improvement theory offered new ways of thinking about that question. I became more concerned with whether or not the clinician's decisions, even if properly learned, were implemented.

Gradually, I focused my knowledge of clinical algorithms on their relationship with clinical guidelines, and my interest in clinical decision making shifted to a preoccupation with clinical decision implementation. Three years later, in 1989, I came to Boston as the Harvard Community Health Plan resident scholar to work on the problem of clinical algorithm reproducibility. By that time interest in clinical guidelines was intense, and people would interrupt my attempts to define algorithms by reassuring me that they were quite familiar with them.

But more than any other single factor, it was helping Larry Gottlieb to create the Institute for Healthcare Improvement course called "Designing Care" that locked in my focus on guideline implementation. First given in the summer of 1990, "Designing Care" was the first course we know to have been aimed at clinicians and to have attempted to teach how to both develop and implement clinical practice guidelines. Over the first 10 course offerings, between 1990 and 1995, more than 500 clinician and administrator participants in the course showed us how to move from emphasizing design to the systematic approach to implementation advocated in this book.

Today, guidelines have become a ubiquitous feature of the clinical care landscape, and my friend Yitzhak is quite familiar with their origins, their potential effects, and their dangers. But he senses that using guidelines is a tricky business. As Avi Porat, another of my colleagues, put it, from the perspective of a sophisticated clinical epidemiologist internist who still spends much time caring for patients and has implemented many guidelines, you don't get three strikes in the guideline business. If you antagonize or threaten a few clinicians sufficiently when trying to implement your first guideline, you are out.

This book was first conceived of by Shan Cretin in 1995. She suggested that the Institute for Healthcare Improvement's "Designing Care" course, taught over 6 years to over 500 clinicians and administrators from all over the United States and abroad, should be turned into a self-learning book. By then, Shan had helped me and Nancy Sokol, an internist and a former associate director of Harvard Community Health Plan's clinical guidelines program, shift the "Designing Care" course to focus much more on implementation. We decided that the book would naturally focus on implementation but would also make available the systematic approach to guideline development that originated at the Center for Medical Decision Making at Ben Gurion University in Israel and in the powerful, groundbreaking guidelines program led by Larry Gottlieb at

Harvard Community Health Plan (now Harvard Pilgrim Health Care). When I began writing in September 1996, it became clear to me that two sorts of expertise would enhance our presentation: the evidence-based approach to guideline development and hands-on experience with guideline program development. Bob Fletcher, the well-known clinical epidemiologist, internist, and former co-editor of the *Annals of Internal Medicine,* not only provided the evidence-based expertise but also brought to his chapter a wealth of experience in attempting to apply these techniques as chairman of guideline development committees at the Agency for Health Care Policy and Research. We were also fortunate to find two groups with extensive experience in different kinds of guideline program development: Dennis Tolsma and Carole Gardner from Kaiser Permanente, Georgia; and Rita Grossman, Charlie Homer, and Don Goldmann from Children's Hospital, Boston. What unifies the authors is that they have all taught or learned about guidelines together at one time or another.

ACKNOWLEDGMENTS

This book got started because of Shan Cretin's suggestion that we turn the "Designing Care" course into a teaching book. Don Berwick and Maureen Bisognano and the Institute for Healthcare Improvement family gave the project a strong push by providing me with support and protected time to write. Audrey Kaufman at AHA Press was as understanding as a senior editor can possibly be while we waited many extra months until all outstanding chapters were received and edited. Strong patient support flowed from Ateret, Mon, and Keshet—my fiercely independent daughters; Adar and Ohr—my pathfinding sons; Lila and Naama—my eloquent daughters-in-law; and Adinah—my constant, feisty wife.

The authors would not have been able to complete their work on this book without huge amounts of editing, typing, and technical assistance from Nurit Barak and Hadar Ben-Shabbat at the Center for Medical Decision Making at Ben-Gurion University of the Negev in Israel and the steady, guiding discipline of Ulka Patel at AHA Press. To all these wonderful people, to many other silent contributors who gave their suggestions and ideas, and to Irene Sotiroff for taking over so smoothly in the stretch, my heartfelt thanks.

Carmi Z. Margolis

Reference

1. J. E. Wennberg and A. Gittelsohn, "Variations in Medical Care among Small Areas," *Sci. Am.* 246 (1982): 120–34.

INTRODUCTION

This book offers a systematic approach to guideline implementation that developed from 10 years of extensive consulting and implementation experience. This approach is based on understanding what clinical guidelines are, how they work, and how implementation techniques that have proved effective in other areas can be used to help implement them. We know that this way of analyzing and developing and implementing guidelines will help anyone use clinical practice guidelines more effectively.

Moreover, this book not only tries to present logical arguments and data but it also aims to teach. We have chosen three techniques to help you, the reader, to feel that you come away from reading any part of the book with knowledge or techniques you can use. First, we have used questions and answers within the text rather than limiting ourselves to plain prose. Second, larger questions are presented as problems for the reader to solve, and solutions are then proposed by the authors. Third, real case scenarios of guideline implementation have been used repeatedly to enable readers to imagine their way through a very lifelike simulation of using guidelines.

INTENDED USERS AND SETTINGS

The authors of this book attempt to explain how to implement clinical practice guidelines effectively in order to help guideline users at any level—whether they are top administrators or line (or even solo!) clinicians—get their job done. The four main groups of users that we have worked with are as follows:

1. Clinicians and clinician administrators, including physicians, nurses, mental health professionals, physical therapists, etc.

2. Medical care administrators, from practice managers up the line to chief executive officers
3. Care policy professionals
4. Health services evaluators and researchers

Health care settings in which guidelines may be implemented are varied and include the following:

- An individual patient
- A practice
- A hospital service
- A group of patients across services and/or practices

Guidelines may also be implemented in educational settings, including medical school courses in clinical judgment or on clerkships, handbooks for residents, and continuing medical education courses.

ORGANIZATION OF THE BOOK

There has been much confusion about how to conceptualize clinical practice guidelines and their use. What is a guideline? How does it work, both from a logical point of view and from a practical point of view when guiding clinical decision making? How do you design and develop a guideline? What is the relationship between developing a valid guideline and implementing it? How does a guideline relate to clinical learning? Can you modify a valid guideline to suit local conditions, or must it be left as is? What is the relationship between quality improvement and clinical guidelines? Conflicting answers have been given to these questions. Even more confusing, pieces of answers may agree, while other parts do not. Frequently, however, these basic questions are addressed almost not at all and guidelines are treated as tools that have to be used to improve quality or cut cost.

Our premise is that because a clinical practice guideline is a conceptual tool, only by understanding what a guideline is—its advantages and limitations—can one optimize guideline use. Above all, we must keep in mind that a practice guideline, even if it is not explicit, frequently guides the cognitive process of clinical decision making. Unlike theoretical cognitive processes, however, clinical decisions must be not only thought about but also acted upon.

This book is organized according to the conceptual framework on which the authors base their understanding of the use of clinical practice guidelines. This framework is illustrated by the guidelines bi-cycle shown in figure FM-1. The figure shows two guideline cycles: the development cycle and the implementation cycle.

FIGURE FM-1. The Guidelines Bi-cycle

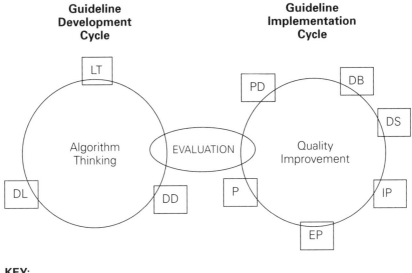

KEY:

DB = Detect Barriers
DD = Design and Development
DL = Dissemination and Learning
DS = Develop Supports
EP = Evaluation Plan

IP = Implementation Plan
LT = Local Tailoring
P = Pilot
PD = Project Design

The development cycle includes the following three complex steps that are facilitated by algorithmic thinking:

1. Design and development: This consists of three key activities—gathering and analyzing the evidence for practicing in a particular way, drafting and redrafting a logically clear and easily communicated guideline, and subjecting guideline drafts to consensus processing.
2. Dissemination and learning: This can be viewed either as the outcome of the guideline development process or as the initial implementation step. However, since it provides the most immediate feedback for revising the guideline, we view it as closely related to development.
3. Local tailoring: This is the final development step, or the initial implementation step. Once tailoring has been accomplished, implementation can proceed.

These steps may be taken in any sort of guideline work, whether it involves developing professional society guidelines, tailoring national ones, or designing a dissemination and learning program for a professional society or a health maintenance organization.

The guideline implementation cycle consists of a quality improvement cycle of six complex steps (figure FM-1), which can be linked to the guideline development cycle right after the local tailoring step, as follows:

1.   Design project
2.   Detect barriers
3.   Develop nonclinical infrastructure supports
4.   Write implementation plan
5.   Write evaluation plan
6.   Run the pilot

These steps should work similarly for implementing a health maintenance organization chest pain guideline or a national immunization guideline. As you can see, the implementation cycle recalls steps of the guideline development cycle. Implementation, like guideline development, involves defining the problem or project, developing or at least choosing a specific guideline, and using it conceptually. The main difference is that when we embark on implementation we must design the nonclinical infrastructure of care so that it enables the clinical guideline to be operationalized. It is the implementation cycle that links guidelines to quality improvement methods and enables us to develop systematic methods for improving clinical quality. Finally, continuous evaluation, like the chain of a bicycle, drives the guideline development and implementation cycles through repeated rounds of modification and improvement.

Chapter 1 presents the basic concepts that enable us to think with guidelines, to define the logic engines called "clinical algorithms" that drive guidelines, and to solve problems with them. Chapter 2 discusses how to choose a clinical guideline project, develop high-quality guidelines, and critique and modify existing guidelines. It also explains how to use nominal group process and the Delphi process to reach consensus on guidelines. Chapter 3 describes how to evaluate and include scientific evidence in the writing of guidelines. Chapter 4 discusses the mechanics of disseminating guidelines, as well as problems and issues involved in learning how to use clinical algorithms. Chapter 5 deals with tailoring guidelines to meet the specific needs of the clinician and the area in which they will be used. Chapter 6 focuses on the implementation of an individual guideline in a pratice setting. In addition to offering strategies for combatting clinician and administrative resistance to guideline implementation, it looks at the role of implementation in the quality improvement process. Chapter 7 explores a method for evaluating and monitoring guidelines. Chapter 8 shifts from discussing how to use guidelines to illustrating successful attempts to set up guideline programs at two different types of institutions: a large health maintenance organization and a major teaching hospital. Finally, there are two appendixes. Appendix A provides an exercise that recaps the implementation process from start to finish. Appendix B contains the answers to the questions and exercises at the back of the individual chapters.

So read the book by all means, but realize that it is meant to be not so much chewed and digested, as Francis Bacon said, but rather to be played with and learned from.

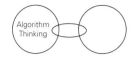

1

Solving Clinical Problems Using Clinical Algorithms

Carmi Z. Margolis, MD, MA

This chapter defines "clinical algorithms" as the logic engines that drive clinical practice guidelines and examines the effect of clinical algorithm use on clinical thinking.

CONCERNS AND QUESTIONS ABOUT CLINICAL ALGORITHMS

In 1971, Franz Ingelfinger wrote an editorial in the *New England Journal of Medicine* called "Algorithms, Anyone?" in which he warned that clinical algorithms have the potential to automate clinical thinking and abolish the art of tailoring decisions to patients' needs.[1]

Sounding his alarm in response to a report by the clinicians and decision-making experts C. H. Sox, H. C. Sox, and R. K. Tompkins of a successful clinical algorithm training system for physician extenders,[2] Ingelfinger foreshadowed many of the concerns that J. P. Kassirer and R. L. Kopelman, experts in medical decision making and experienced internists, would voice 17 years later,[3] as guidelines and algorithms were becoming familiar concepts. Starting from Ingelfinger's view of the algorithm as a prescription, they focus on the inherently rigid nature of clinical algorithms, the lack of a rigorous, standardized methodology to develop them, the danger of missing patients' problems not covered by the algorithm, and the lack of studies demonstrating their effectiveness.

In sharp contrast to the view that a clinical algorithm is nothing more than a step-by-step prescription, A. R. Feinstein in 1974 wrote that flowchart algorithms provide the clinician with language, heretofore unavailable, to "specify the flow of logic in his reasoning."[4] Though perhaps surprising at first, this view of algorithms as both powerful and potentially flexible aids to thinking also has intuitive appeal. Most of us realize that chess computer algorithms can challenge grandmasters,[5] and Caduceus algorithms for internal medicine diagnosis solve the *New England Journal of Medicine* CPCs.[6] Lev Landa, the Russian proponent of algorithms for teaching,[7] as well as psychologists B. H. Lewis and G. Pask in England,[8] insisted 25 years ago that the solution to any problem can be taught more effectively if the problem can be analyzed algorithmically. Edward Fretkin, the self-taught computer genius who became a professor without a bachelor's degree at the Massachusetts Institute of Technology, has even hinted that there might be a godlike universal algorithm that governs all physics.[9]

Which of these contradictory views of algorithms in general, and clinical ones in particular, is correct? Are they flexible and powerful or anticreative, automatic, and rigid? By examining the following basic questions regarding the nature and use of algorithms, I propose to show that, in fact, both of these apparently irreconcilable views are correct:

- What is an algorithm?
- Is a clinical algorithm a mathematical algorithm?
- What are the uses of clinical algorithms?
- Do algorithms and protocols limit clinical thinking?
- What is a clinical practice guideline?
- How are practice guidelines related to clinical algorithms?
- Will practice guidelines limit, or even make dangerous, the art of tailoring decisions to individual patients?
- What are the main characteristis of a high-quality clinical practice guideline?

The following subsections examine these questions in depth.

What Is an Algorithm?

Invented by the Persian mathematician al-Chaforisme in the ninth century, an algorithm is a step-by-step approach to solving a problem that usually involves conditional logic.[10] However, although many of us could come up with a similar definition, and we all learned to do arithmetic problems using variations on al-Chaforisme's original arithmetic algorithms, the definition of an algorithm is frequently confused with the format in which it is presented.

Exhibit 1-1 and figure 1-1 show two examples of algorithm formats. The recipe listed in exhibit 1-1 is an algorithm for preparing Sabbath saffron rice, and the flowchart in figure 1-1 is an algorithm for guessing in fewer than five guesses the day of the month someone was born. Lists and flowcharts are not necessarily algorithms, but algorithms might be presented in list, flowchart, or prose format. Each of these formats has a different main use. List algorithms are most effective for directing actions, be they for computers or nurse practitioners, while flowchart or map algorithms are more effective than prose for teaching decision making involving complex sequences of dependent decisions.

Lighting the definition of an algorithm from another angle, the concept of algorithm parsimony or efficiency implies that there is always more than one way to define an algorithm and that some ways are more efficient, though not necessarily more effective, than others. Version 2 of the birthday guessing game algorithm (figure 1-2) has fewer steps and is thus more efficient than version 1, but would be less effective than version 1 for teaching a child the game (in fact, version 1 was designed by a mother/child team).[11]

Is a Clinical Algorithm a Mathematical Algorithm?

Viewed as a step-by-step approach to solving a defined clinical problem that involves conditional logic, a clinical algorithm shares the basic characteristics of a mathematical algorithm, but is not actually a mathematical algorithm. Rather, it belongs to the set of algorithms first used shortly after the first computer was built in 1945 and that I call "the practical algorithm."

EXHIBIT 1-1. Part of a Recipe for Sabbath Saffron Rice

Sabbath Saffron Rice

Ingredients:
1. 1.5 cups long-grain rice
2. 3 cups hot broth
3. 6 tablespoons oil from a roast

Instructions:
1. Place rice in a saucepan with the oil and cook.
2. When rice makes a sharp, dry noise (c. 3 minutes), add 1 cup of hot broth and cook over high heat for 5 minutes.

etc.

From E. S. Machlin, *The Classic Cuisine of the Italian Jews* (New York: Dodd, Mead & Co., 1981), p. 116.

FIGURE 1-1. Birthday Guessing Game Algorithm—Version 1

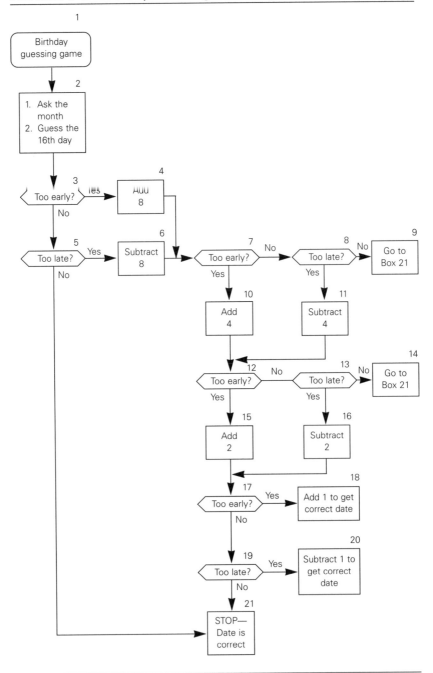

Reprinted, with permission, from *Designing Care Coursebook*, published by the Institute for Healthcare Improvement, Boston, © 1991–1996.

FIGURE 1-2. Birthday Guessing Game Algorithm—Version 2

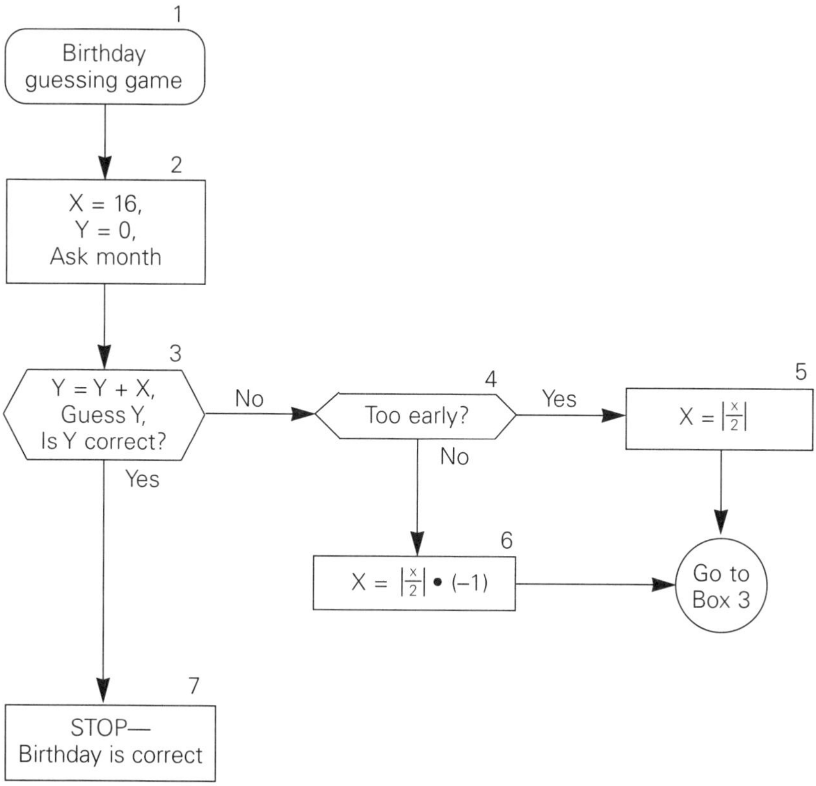

Typical characteristics of Feinstein's practical traffic light algorithm (figure 1-3) highlight the differences between practical and mathematical algorithms. Notice that certain obvious aspects of the problem of traversing an intersection, such as dealing with a broken light, a policeman, or a turn, are not dealt with in the traffic light algorithm. Practical algorithms characteristically do not define all situations implied by the problem definition. They compensate for this in part by leaving fuzzy definitions and endings, such as "cogent reason for running the light" and "make new decision if situation changes," that rely on the algorithm user's judgment. Underlying these special characteristics of the practical algorithm is the unpredictable nature of the problem it purports to solve. In contrast to the finite 31 possible solutions to the birthday guessing game, it is not possible to predict, even using a much more complex traffic light algorithm, all the situations that might arise when approaching a traffic light.

FIGURE 1-3. Traffic Light Algorithm

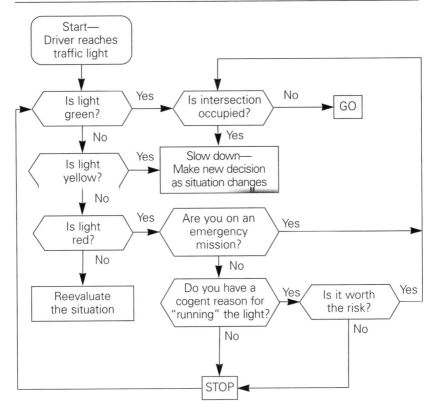

Reprinted, with permission, from A.R. Feinstein, "An Analysis of Diagnostic Reasoning: III. The Construction of Clinical Algorithms," *Yale Journal of Biological Medicine,* New Haven, CT, © 1974; 47: 5–32.

Clearly, variations between patients are even more unpredictable than variations between intersections, and clinical algorithms therefore require user judgment. Practical algorithms, drawn as flowcharts with pictures at key decision points, became known in the graphics literature as job performance aids. They were already used by the U.S. Army in the 1940s to teach recruits complicated tasks, such as fixing an airplane aileron or tuning a pneumatic controller.[12] W. J. Tuddenham, chairman of the department of radiology at the University of Pennsylvania, designed a flowchart algorithm with pictures for teaching radiology technicians how to diagnose a barium enema. This first clinical algorithm I know of to be published in English, is an example of a job performance aid type of practical algorithm.[13]

What Are the Uses of Clinical Algorithms?

Like other practical algorithms, clinical algorithms have three main uses:

1. To analyze the approach to solving a clinical problem
2. To teach the approach
3. To guide action

To demonstrate for yourself the teaching advantages of the flowchart algorithm, try to calculate your capital gains tax using B. N. Lewis and J. A. Cook's quote from the British income tax instructions that appears in exhibit 1-2.[14] Give up? In figure 1-4, you will find a flowchart, or algorithm map, that contains the identical content, but enables a user with a few basic definitions (similar to the ingredients in a recipe or patient data in a pharyngitis algorithm) to calculate capital gains tax within a few minutes.

Characteristics of the Algorithm Map   Two features of the flowchart or algorithm map make it useful for describing decision making:

1. Decisions and their sequencing are clearly defined in boxes and are linked by directional lines.
2. The flowchart graphic presents a picture of the problem analysis that prose, with its stylized use of the space between words, sentences, and lines, does not allow.

EXHIBIT 1-2. A Quote from British Income Tax Instructions

If the asset consists of stocks or shares which have values quoted on a stock exchange (see also paragraph G below), or unit trust units whose values are regularly quoted, the gain or loss (subject to expenses) accruing after 6 April 1965 is the difference between the amount you received on disposal and the market value on 6 April 1965—except that in the case of a gain where the actual cost of the asset was higher than the value at 6 April 1965, the chargeable gain is the excess of the amount you received on disposal over the original cost or acquisition price; and in the case of a loss, where the actual cost of the asset was lower than the value at 6 April 1965, the allowable loss is the excess of the original cost or acquisition price over the amount received on disposal.

If the substitution of original cost for the value at 6 April 1965 turns a gain into a loss, or a loss into a gain, there is, for the purpose of tax, no chargeable gain or allowable loss.

Reprinted from *International Journal of Man-Machine Studies,* 1, B. N. Lewis and J. A. Cook, "Toward a Theory of Telling," 129–176, 1969, by permission of the publisher, Academic Press Limited, London.

FIGURE 1-4. Capital Gains Tax Algorithm

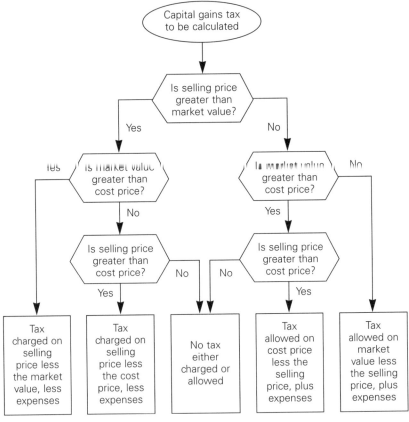

Reprinted from *International Journal of Man-Machine Studies,* 1, B. N. Lewis and J. A. Cook, "Toward a Theory of Telling," 129–176, 1969, by permission of the publisher, Academic Press Limited, London.

Feinstein saw in these characteristics of the algorithm flowchart or map the special language that had been lacking to describe and teach clinical practice. C. Z. Margolis and colleagues used this charting or mapping to analyze the logic of clinical management, and showed in a prospective controlled trial that medical students and residents learn more effectively and efficiently from clinical algorithms than from prose how to manage fever and meningitis in children.[15]

List Format Algorithms Mapping problem approaches, however, does not insure that, or document whether, the map has been used. List format algorithms such as the U.S. income tax return (for example, Form 1040) lend themselves more readily to this prospective use of algorithms.

An example of a list format algorithm that applies to health care institutions is the clinical protocol. Clinical protocols, or protocol charts (exhibit 1-3), are lists of instructions for collecting and using clinical data that appear on an encounter form and are wired conditionally according to the logic of the clinical algorithm (figure 1-5). Protocols have been used with much success to guide and document clinical care by nurse practitioners, physician extenders, and physicians.[16-20]

An example of a flowchart format algorithm used to evaluate the process of health care is a criteria map. A criteria map is a clinical algorithm application closely related to protocol charts that enables a trained technician to perform reliable and valid medical record audits according to conditional criteria (figure 1-6). Compared to the traditional medical record audit, which uses criteria lists in which the items are grouped without being arranged according to conditional logic, the criteria map audit has been shown to produce more believable scores and even to predict outcome.[21]

Do Algorithms and Protocols Limit Clinical Thinking?

Ingelfinger as well as Kassirer and Kopelman assumed that the answer to this question is yes. If so, then one would expect protocol systems to succeed only when used by physician extenders (assistants), whose clinical knowledge base and problem-solving potential is limited. However, physicians have also used protocols successfully.[22] Is it plausible to assume that a physician's decision making is limited by an algorithm or that a physician extender's is extended by one? How is this conceptual tool used to solve medical problems? Analyzing the attempt of a group of physicians to implement protocols will help clarify the answer to this question.

Physician Attempts to Implement Protocols Experienced pediatricians once began to use the computerized flowchart protocols that they designed themselves to guide the process of caring for common problems.[22] Within a month, however, they became irritated with the tediousness of checking off, patient by patient, the step-by-step protocol charts, and refused to continue using the protocols. In reviewing this experiment, one cannot assume either that the algorithm logic behind the protocols or the checklist format were unacceptable, since the pediatricians themselves developed the algorithms, and the flowchart format used to record patient visits on the computer did not have the off-putting aspect of a checklist. What caused the pediatricians to discontinue using the algorithms was their impatience at having to spend unnecessary time recording every step of a thinking process they knew intimately and could shortcut successfully.

EXHIBIT 1-3.   Male Genitourinary Protocol (11/75)

Chief complaint(s)

	Yes	No	SUBJECTIVE	Duration
1			Urethral discharge	_____
2			Painful urination	_____
3			Urgency/frequency	_____
4			Any duration greater than one month	
5			New pain/swelling in joints	
6			Painful scrotum/ testicle	
7			New rash/ sores present now	
8			Chills/fever	
9			Here for Rx of + GC cult	DxGC

	Yes	No	OBJECTIVE	
10			Temperature greater than 100 degrees	_____
11			Conjunctivitis/ photophobia	
12			Enlarged inguinal lymph nodes	
13			Urethral warts	
14			Other warts	Remove or refer
15			Genital rash/lesions	Examine for lice
16			Genital itch	
17			Lice found	Rx Kwell

Reprinted, with permission, from The Beth Israel Hospital Association, Boston, and Massachusetts Institute of Technology, Cambridge, 1975–HEW Contract No. HSM 110-73-335.

Pediatricians who were expert at common problem management could no more tolerate being forced to move stepwise through algorithms for managing common problems than can a professor of mathematics be forced to write the addition algorithm each time he has to add seven and three.

FIGURE 1-5. Male Genitourinary Problems Algorithm

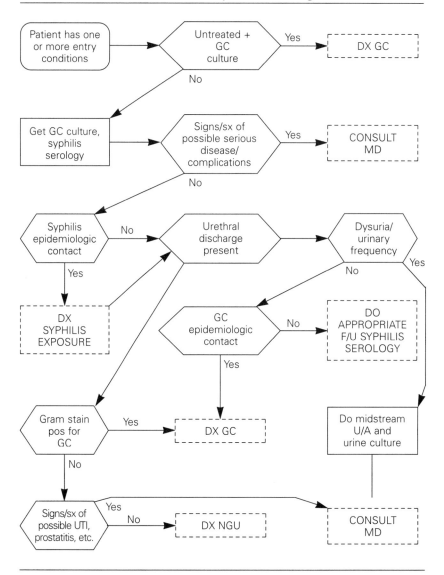

Reprinted, with permission, from A. Komaroff, *Common Acute Problems,* published by Little, Brown and Co., Boston, 1977.

FIGURE 1-6. Abstraction Map for Pneumonia—a Part of a Conditional Criteria Audit of Acute Pneumonia in Children

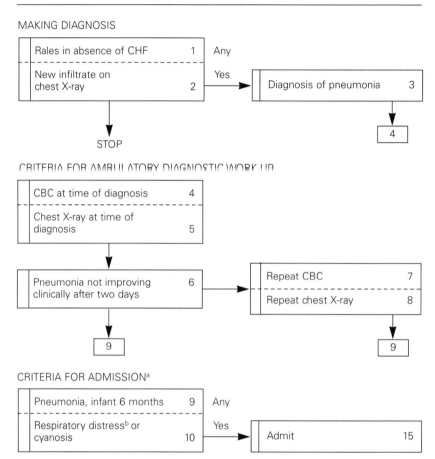

MAKING DIAGNOSIS

CRITERIA FOR AMBULATORY DIAGNOSTIC WORK-UP

CRITERIA FOR ADMISSION[a]

[a] Two of the six criteria used are presented in this figure.

[b] Respiratory distress = respiratory rate 50% normal for age; moderate retractions (suprasternal, substernal, or intercostal; air hunger)

Reprinted, with permission, from *Solving Common Pediatric Problems: an Algorithm Approach,* published by The Solomon Press, New York, © 1981.

Physician Extender Attempts to Implement Protocols Physician extenders or nurse practitioners, although lacking sophisticated basic science knowledge, do not have a different algorithm learning psychology. Investigators who have trained mid-level practitioners using clinical algorithms or protocols have observed repeatedly that after the initial months of training, when encounter forms serve as behavioral feedback loops for reinforcing algorithm learning, mid-level practitioners become resistant to filling out protocols, even though they continue to practice according to algorithm logic. Similarly, while the pediatricians were still using their computerized flowchart protocols, the process of care changed from pre-protocol care to the care process specified in the flow-charts, much as one would expect of mid-level practitioner care.[22] One concludes that care provided by experienced clinicians should be related closely to the guiding algorithm, but does not always have to be thought about step-by-step, in the way that a computer solves a mathematical problem.

Inducers to Successful Protocol Implementation Henderson and colleagues have demonstrated in a controlled trial not only that experi-enced clinicians will use computerized clinical algorithms to care for patients with adult respiratory distress syndrome,[23] but, as was shown in an earlier experiment with emergency medical technicians using arrhythmia algorithms,[24] that algorithm-treated patients also had signifi-cantly lower mortality. The investigators point out that practitioner unfa-miliarity with the intricacies of managing these patients, conducting weekly updatings of algorithm logic by a clinician/programmer team, careful use of clinician consensus to develop the algorithms, and collect-ing ongoing feedback to practitioners on patient outcome were all pow-erful inducers to successful protocol implementation by physicians.

Human versus Computer Use of Algorithms A closer look at human as opposed to computer use of algorithms enables us to rethink the concept that algorithms limit thinking. Arithmetic algorithms limit one's thinking to solving arithmetic problems. However, once their step-by-step procedures have been memorized and internalized, they can be traversed instantly and can increase one's ability to solve a wide range of mathematical problems. Solving many mathematical problems requires the solver to know how to both solve arithmetic problems and recognize when arithmetic is not needed to solve a problem. Similarly, a diagnos-tic anemia algorithm limits the clinicians' thinking not by restricting it, but rather by focusing it on a stepwise approach to diagnosing anemia. Like the arithmetic algorithm that will not solve algebra problems, an anemia algorithm will not diagnose the cause of respiratory failure or fever. Unlike the arithmetic algorithm that always solves arithmetic prob-lems, the anemia algorithm will not apply to all anemia patients, since some of them will not fit the algorithm, either because they have an asso-ciated problem, say fever or seizures, or because of some other special patient or environmental characteristic. However, the anemia algorithm might still help to diagnose these patients by clarifying that they require a different algorithm or some other problem-solving approach. Moreover, the anemia algorithm can be fit together with a different algorithm to diagnose a patient with several problems or with a complex problem, in the same way that the addition algorithm is used to add similar algebraic symbols to help solve an algebra problem.

In summary, the following general process of clinical algorithm learning has been observed in clinicians at all levels of sophistication:

1. Clinicians are more motivated to learn from, and will adhere more closely to, clinical algorithms concerning problems with which they are unfamiliar.

2. Once they learn an algorithm thoroughly, clinicians will begin to take shortcuts through it and will resist following or documenting their path through the clinical algorithm.

3. Using a clinical algorithm will assist in solving problems not related to the clinical algorithm, either by indicating what the problem is not, or by combining the clinical algorithm or part of it with another clinical algorithm or another problem-solving technique. An implication of this observation is that cognitive care provided by physicians ought to derive from their sophisticated basic science knowledge and should include writing clinical algorithms. They should practice solving complex problems that require either merging clinical algorithms (or parts of clinical algorithms) or are not amenable to algorithmic solution.[25, 26]

What Is a Clinical Practice Guideline?

Two main perspectives of clinical practice guidelines are the viewpoint of clinical learning and that of clinical work. From a clinical learning perspective, clinical practice guidelines are tools that might help you solve clinical problems. From a clinical work perspective, clinical practice guidelines are processes of clinical work that you must carry out in order to care for a patient's problem. Each of these ways of thinking about clinical practice guidelines has different implications, and different advantages and disadvantages. Learning both of these concepts, like any journey, starts at home. Conceptually, home is the definition of a clinical practice guideline, or knowing what it is and how it works.

A useful definition of a clinical practice guideline, similar to that proposed by the Institute of Medicine, is as follows: all the information relevant to a diagnostic and therapeutic approach to the solution and care of a patient's medical problem. However, this definition explains little about how a guideline helps the clinician solve the patient's problem. To use guidelines effectively, rather than having them stand between us and the patient like any unfamiliar diagnostic test or therapy, we must learn to understand and use the clinical algorithm embedded in every guideline. Like a conceptual locomotive pulling an information train, this clinical algorithm is the logic engine that makes the clinical practice guideline go.

How Are Practice Guidelines Related to Clinical Algorithms?

Intense guideline development efforts by the government, the health care industry, and the health care professions over the past eight years provide examples of the mechanisms that turn algorithms into guideline logic engines. Quantitative, probabilistic methods proposed by D. M. Eddy, the medical decision-making, policy, and guidelines expert, for deriving guideline decisions from empirical data, such as metanalysis and decision analysis, have been contrasted with deterministic clinical algorithms that are sometimes portrayed as inferior and lacking in validity.[27] Such a superficial comparison, however, misses the point. Evidence-based techniques and algorithms are in fact complementary, since a successful quantitative analysis leads inevitably to establishing some sort of formal rule or clinical algorithm.

The expense of quantitative methods in time and money and their focus on single decisions precludes developing rules or algorithms for much of medicine in the near future. Guideline development techniques involving consensus and qualitative literature review will be much needed. Published consensus guidelines, such as the practice policies of the American Academy of Pediatrics that have gained wide acceptance over the years, might contain facts and principles best described in prose. However, the central recommendations, sometimes buried but always there, consist of conditional stepwise algorithmic rules that would be more understandable and usable if presented as algorithm maps or flowcharts. Both these methods, evidence-based and consensus-based rule derivation, are used to derive a common conceptual tool, the clinical algorithm, that embodies guideline logic and drives guideline use in practice.

A more useful contrast between much investigated, evidence-based guideline derivation methods and algorithmic guideline logic rules is to define their interdependent relationship clearly—the relation between the evidence that underpins a clinical practice guideline and guideline logic (discussed in chapter 3). The guideline's algorithmic nature and even the consensus process itself has hardly been investigated. Such research would concentrate on questions relating to the nature of consensus, how much of a guideline must be based on consensus, and on methods for defining guideline reproducibility, reliability, and validity.

Will Practice Guidelines Limit or Even Make Dangerous the Art of Tailoring Decisions to Individual Patients (That Is, the Art of Medical Practice)?

This question recalls the essence of Ingelfinger's reservation about algorithms. Our answer is that guidelines should limit, not clinical thinking, but rather the inappropriately wide range of approaches to a clinical problem that lies at the root of government and health care industry pre-occupation with unacceptable variation in quality. Guidelines will make practice dangerous only if they are viewed as mathematical algorithms that can be applied automatically and would thus limit the clinician's judgment regarding how and when to apply the guideline. But insisting that guideline use restricts freer thinking makes no more sense than saying that airline pilots are restricted by protocols for flying a plane, or that pilots would be more likely to adapt to unusual situations if they did not use any protocols or checklists at all. As we have tried to show, rather than straitjacketing the clinician and endangering the patient, the algorithmic part of a guideline should facilitate the art of making specific clinical decisions and improve the quality of practice by making it explicit.

The real difficulties with using guidelines are as follows:

- Improper development
- Failure to take into account rationally justifiable local variations in practice, environment, or populations
- Shortcutting by skilled practitioners

These implementation problems, in turn, are mainly due to not applying quality improvement techniques to the problem of redesigning the nonclinical, essential infrastructure of clinical care. A key reciprocal relationship is that just as clinical practice guidelines provide someone attempting to improve clinical quality with a clinical process description, so does quality improvement technique provide clinical practice guideline implementors with the means to effective implementation. The means for effective implementation—that is, quality improvement techniques—are as follows: emphasis on team problem solving that considers administrative as well as clinical aspects of care; emphasis on analysis of the care system as key to clinical quality improvement; and, most important, emphasis on the customer's (patient's) perspective.

These real difficulties are frequently amenable to the methods this book attempts to teach for developing, disseminating, tailoring, and implementing quality clinical practice guidelines. Let us consider what a quality guideline is.

What Are the Main Characteristics of a High-Quality Clinical Practice Guideline?

In 1990, Field and Lohr proposed the now commonplace, nine-part, Institute of Medicine (IOM) definition of a good clinical practice guideline.[28] They wrote that good guidelines are characterized by the following:

1. Validity (improves health)
2. Reliability (different users use it with the same results)
3. Reproducibility (a kind of reliability, independent experts generate similar guidelines)
4. Applicability (population it refers to is defined)
5. Flexibility (population it does not apply to is defined)
6. Clarity
7. Scheduled review
8. Good documentation
9. Multidisciplinary review

We do not disagree with any of these good guideline characteristics, but we feel that they can be reduced and clarified. A high-quality clinical practice guideline must minimally demonstrate three main characteristics.

First, it must be clear. Clarity has been de-emphasized in much guideline work, but it cannot be overemphasized. Since clinical practice guidelines are powered by clinical algorithm logic engines that might be of considerable complexity, learning to think flexibly and appropriately with clinical practice guidelines depends on algorithm and guideline clarity. We have stressed that clarity in turn depends in large part on graphic techniques for making the guideline algorithm explicit and clear.

Second, it must be useable. Even if the guideline is backed by evidence and is reliable (that is, different users use it with similar results), it must have been tailored to local conditions and be accompanied by plans for redesigning administrative processes to enable its use in an actual care setting. (Tailoring guidelines is discussed in chapter 5.) Although the IOM definition makes little mention of this issue, and though it depends largely on factors external to the guideline, we are convinced that usability is an essential guideline quality. Consider, then, that you cannot determine whether a generic guideline, be it one by the Agency for Health Care Policy and Research or one by the American College of Physicians, has all the characteristics of a good guideline, since a generic version can no more be assessed for usability than for scheduled review.

Third, it must improve care and, hopefully, health. We deliberately present this guideline quality last, not because it is least important, but because the first two qualities need to be emphasized. Guideline efficacy, or the potential to improve care, derives from its validity, which in turn derives from the quality of the evidence and the strength of the consensus on which it rests.

The aim of the rest of this book is to provide you with the tools to use quality clinical practice guidelines. Let us begin by discussing the first step in the guideline development cycle, guideline development.

QUESTIONS FOR STUDY

1. What is a clinical algorithm?
2. What are three differences between practical and mathematical algorithms?
3. Define clinical practice guideline.
4. What is the relationship between a clinical practice guideline and its clinical algorithm?
5. What is a job performance aid?
6. What is the relationship between an algorithm and a flowchart?
7. What are three other formats for presenting clinical algorithms, and how are they used?
8. What are the main uses of a clinical algorithm?
9. Do clinical algorithms limit (decrease flexibility) clinical thinking?
10. What are three main characteristics of a quality guideline?

The answers to these questions can be found in Appendix B.

References and Notes

1. F. Ingelfinger, "Algorithms, Anyone?" *N. Engl. J. Med.* 288 (1973): 847–8.

2. C. H. Sox, H. C. Sox, and R. K. Tompkins, "The Training of Physician's Assistants: The Use of a Clinical Algorithm System for Patient Care, Audit of Performance and Education," *N. Engl. J. Med.* 288 (1973): 818–24.

3. J. P. Kassirer and R. L. Kopelman, "Diagnosis and Decision by Algorithms," *Hosp. Prac.* 23 (1990): 23–31.

4. A. R. Feinstein, "An Analysis of Diagnostic Reasoning: III. The Construction of Clinical Algorithms," *Yale J. Bio. Med.* 47 (1974): 5–32.

5. H. R. Lewis and C. H. Papadimitriou, "The Efficiency of Algorithms," *Sci. Am.* 238, no. 1 (1978): 96–109.

6. R. A. Miller, H. E. Pople, and J. D. Myers, "Internist-I, An Experimental Computer Base Diagnostic Consultant for General Internal Medicine," *N. Engl. J. Med.* 307 (1982): 68–476.

7. L. N. Landa, *Instructional Regulation and Control: Cybernetics, Algorithmization, and Heuristics in Education* (Englewood Cliffs, NJ: Educational Technology Publications, 1976).

8. B. H. Lewis and G. Pask, *Case Studies in the Use of Algorithms* (London: Pergamon Press, 1967).

9. R. Wright, "Did the Universe Just Happen?" *The Atlantic* 261 (1988): 29–52.

10. "Algorithms," in *Encyclopaedia Britannica, Micropedia* (Chicago: Helen Hemingway Benton, 1979), Vol. 1., p. 239.

11. Dr. Katherine Grimes, personal communication.

12. R. J. Smillie, "Design Strategies for Job Performance Aids," in *Designing Usable Texts,* I. M. Duffy and R. Waller, eds. (New York: Academic Press, 1985).

13. W. J. Tuddenham, "The Use of Logical Flowcharts As an Aid in Teaching Roentgen Diagnosis," *Am. J. Roentgenol.* 102 (1968): 797–803.

14. B. N. Lewis and J. A. Cook, "Toward a Theory of Telling," *Int. J. Man-Machine Studies* 1 (1969): 129–76.

15. C. Z. Margolis, C. D. Cook, N. Barak, A. Adler, A. Geertsma, "Clinical Algorithms Teach Pediatric Decision-making More Effectively Than Prose," *Med. Care* 27 (1989): 576–92.

16. H. C. Sox, "Quality of Patient Care by Nurse Practitioners and Physician's Assistants: A Ten-Year Perspective," *Ann. Intern. Med.* 91 (1979): 459–68.

17. F. P. Wilson, L. O. Wilson, M. F. Wheeler, L. Canales, and R. W. Wood, "Algorithm-Directed Care by Non-Physician Practitioner Data-Gathering Behavior," *Med. Care* 21 (1983): 127–37.

18. D. Wirtschafter, J. T. Carpenter, and E. Mesel, "A Consultant-Extender System for Breast Cancer Adjacent Chemotherapy," *Ann. Int. Med.* 90 (1979): 396–401.

19. C. D. Cook and J. Heidt, *Assuring Quality Out-Patient Care for Children: Guidelines and Management System* (New York: Oxford University Press, 1987).

20. W. H. Frazier and D. A. Brand, "Quality Assessment and the Art of Medicine: The Anatomy of Laceration Care," *Med. Care* 17 (1979): 480–90.

21. S. Greenfield, S. Cretin, L. G. Worthman, "Comparison of a Criteria Map to a Criteria List in Quality of Care Assessment for Patients with Chest Pain: The Relation of Each to Outcome," *Med. Care* 19 (1981): 255–72.

22. C. Z. Margolis, S. Warshawsky, L. Goldman, O. Dagan, D. D. Wirtschafter, and J. S. Pliskin, "Computerized Algorithms and Pediatricians' Management of Common Problems in a Community Clinic," *Acad. Med.* 67 (1992): 282.

23. S. Henderson, T. D. East, A. H. Morris, and R. M. Gardner, "Performance Evaluation of Computerized Clinical Protocols for Management of Arterial Hypoxemia in AIDS Patients," Proceedings, 13th Annual Symposium on Computer Applications in Medical Care, Washington, DC, 1989.

24. G. C. Cayten, G. Oler, and R. S. Staroscik, "Clinical Algorithms for Pre Hospital Cardiac Care," *Med. Care* 21 (1983):147–56.

25. A discussion of other clinical problem-solving methods, such as pattern recognition or Weed's problem-oriented approach, is essential for a more complete understanding of medical problem solving, but is outside the scope of this discussion

26. C. Z. Margolis, "Uses of Clinical Algorithms," *JAMA* 249 (1983): 627–32.

27. D. M. Eddy, "Practice Policies: Where Do They Come From? *JAMA* 263 (1990):1265, 1269, 1272, 1275.

28. M. Y. Field and K. N. Lohr, eds., *Clinical Practice Guidelines: Directions for a New Agency* (Washington, DC: Institute of Medicine, National Academy Press, 1990).

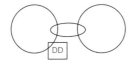

2

Developing and Constructing Practical Guidelines

Carmi Z. Margolis, MD, MA

Three questions face the novice guideline developer embarking on a new project. First, "How do I choose a clinical guideline project?" Second, "once I've chosen a project, how do I develop a quality clinical guideline?" And third, "How do I critique and modify an existing clinical guideline for use in my own setting?" Similar questions continue to irk the experienced implementor.

This chapter is divided into three sections, each of which addresses the questions above. The third section introduces two techniques—nominal group process and the Delphi process—and explains how they can be used to critique and modify practice guidelines.

CHOOSING A GUIDELINE PROJECT

While there are several situations in which you can use a clinical guideline effectively, there is only one situation in which a clinical guideline should not be used, and that is when there is no chance of agreement on the diagnostic and therapeutic approach to a clinical problem. For example, there is no point in writing a clinical guideline for the management of patients with an undiagnosed problem if that problem is not usually seen and is not amenable to a systematic workup (for example, seizures and severe hemolysis in a patient with systemic lupus erythematosis). In 1986, when we began working in Boston on a clinical guideline for osteoporosis, we discovered there was no agreement on how to manage it (in the words of one expert, "Any agreement that there was last year at this time has eroded!") and we scrapped the clinical guideline. In addition, it is not useful to write a clinical guideline recommending therapy that is controversial unless there is a body of evidence to support that therapy and the caveats are clearly explained in an annotation.

However, assuming you are fairly certain that there is general agreement on the approach to managing a certain problem, there are three major reasons for developing and implementing a clinical guideline:

1. To control practice variation
2. To decrease cost
3. To map the approach to an uncommon problem

These three reasons for using clinical guidelines appeal to different user groups. Less experienced users will be more likely to use common problem clinical guidelines that limit practice variation. Very experienced users will prefer to write clinical guidelines for common problems and to use clinical guidelines for rarer problems. Managers will seek out clinical guidelines that correct obvious errors, update practice, or control cost.

Although any of these groups might be motivated to use a clinical guideline for any of the three major reasons, it is important to consider whether experienced practitioners will use a common problem clinical guideline at all. This question will be considered in chapter 6, but a brief answer is that they will if the clinical guideline is unobtrusive. On the other hand, if they are being constantly reminded to do something they are quite familiar with, they might reject documenting or even using the clinical guideline.

Controlling Practice Variation

The most important reason for implementing a guideline is to control practice variation. You might think that when we say "controlling variation" we mean "controlling cost," but in our experience, cutting cost is only one reason for controlling variation. A more compelling reason is improving quality. Consider the following story:

Some years ago, a group of four pediatricians who had worked together for several years felt that they were taking care of common problems in quite different ways.[1] In order to clarify these differences, they spent many hours over a period of two months discussing each of six clinical algorithms on wheezing, gastroenteritis, croup, urinary tract infection, otitis media, and pneumonia. One of several surprises was that two of them were using different antibiotics in a different sequence for otitis media in contrast to the other two. After a long discussion that led to a reexamination of the literature, all four agreed on a consistent sequence of the same antibiotics. The result of all the discussions was a revised set of algorithm maps that represented their own approaches to these six problems.

Skeptical managers, clinical more often than nonclinical ones, will probably balk at this point. They might feel that these pediatricians are not representative. They seem academically oriented or just peculiar. However, we suggest that most well-trained practitioners have learned or developed for themselves consistent approaches to solving many clinical problems. For clinicians, part of the fun of medicine is discussing the reasoning that buttresses these approaches and determining at which points no consistent approach can be defined.

However, the motivation for correcting or updating practice might come from the environment, especially from the patient. Consider this example:

In 1989, Mrs. Severity, a mother and a lawyer, wrote a furious letter implying malpractice to Dr. Harvey, medical director of a large group practice. In it, she explained that she had taken her 11-year-old son, Paul, to the clinic after 24 hours of high fever, shaking chills, and a bad sore throat. The pediatrician took a throat culture, saying that the result would be back within 36 hours, and recommended supportive care with aspirin, fluids, and lozenges. But the result came back positive days later, after the weekend. Meanwhile, Paul was in bed with high fever, chills, and much discomfort for two days after leaving the clinic, until his mother decided to give him penicillin on Sunday night. He was much better by Monday afternoon. Mrs. Severity noted two errors she believed were evidence of incompetence. First, Paul could have been treated while waiting for culture results. Second, the clinic could have done a rapid strep test. Dr. Harvey tended to agree with her first criticism, but was unconvinced that the rapid strep test was cost effective. He consulted us because he wanted to implement a pediatric pharyngitis clinical guideline that would make a clear recommendation regarding use of the rapid strep test. He and his colleagues did go on to develop the clinical guideline, which recommended culturing and treating immediately in a toxic patient with pharyngitis, but did not recommend use of the rapid strep test because of its variable sensitivity. Mrs. Severity did not sue the clinic.

Decreasing Cost

Another cogent reason for implementing a clinical guideline is to decrease cost. For example, introducing a "low back pain" guideline should limit the use of both spine x-rays and computed axial tomography scans, thus reducing cost. Remember, however, that clinical guidelines do not necessarily reduce cost. For example, if someone suffered a blow to the head and was knocked unconscious in 1972 (or in 1998 in a setting with limited facilities such as Lilongwe, the capital city of Malawi, Africa), the emergency room physician, in keeping with accepted practice, would order skull films. As computed axial tomography scans have become available, the clinical guideline has changed to require a computed axial tomography scan for specific clinical indications after head trauma, so that a far more expensive procedure is necessary to assure quality.

Mapping the Approach to an Uncommon Problem

For experienced practitioners, decreasing variation and reducing cost are not the only major reasons for implementing a clinical guideline. Another reason is unfamiliarity with the workup and management of less common clinical problems. While the average primary care internist or family practitioner would prefer writing a chest pain clinical guideline to following one step-by-step (why should he or she follow a systematic approach to solving a clinical problem that he or she is adept at short-cutting?), the same practitioner might be delighted to follow with precision a thyroid nodule clinical guideline if he or she sees such patients only occasionally.

DEVELOPING A QUALITY CLINICAL GUIDELINE

There are three essential elements in a quality guideline: clinical experience, evidence, and consensus. Although it might seem that different groups working in different environments use different strategies, our experience has been that all guideline development strategies are similar in that they contain some or all of the following six steps:

1. Generate/choose the seed algorithm
2. Marshal the evidence
3. Perform consensus processing
4. Write the first revision of the algorithm seed
5. Repeat iterations of steps 3 and 4
6. Produce the penultimate draft

Note that while the last four of the above steps usually occur in the order listed, the first two could certainly be reversed. We chose, however, to present generating/choosing the seed algorithm first, because we feel strongly that this technique enables an experienced clinician to capture best how he or she approaches clinical problem management. Faced with a quality clinical algorithm, many clinicians will respond (even if they disagree with specific points in the algorithm or they feel uncomfortable writing algorithms themselves) that this is the way they think about their work. The clinical algorithm is also an excellent way to get an overview of the key points in management that should be buttressed by evidence. Finally, constructing or analyzing the algorithmic logic that drives a clinical guideline, though it becomes more important as the clinical logic becomes more complex, is the step that is most frequently overlooked in developing a guideline.

Step 1. Generate/Choose the Seed Algorithm

At the present time, managers or clinicians do not usually have to generate a guideline from scratch. Well-documented and -researched guidelines on many of the common primary care problems are easily available. Following are some examples of quality template guidelines:

- Management of pediatric or adult asthma
- Management of chest pain in adults
- General surgery
- Depression managed by primary care practitioners or psychiatrists

The Ben-Gurion University Center for Medical Decision Making has collected many sources of clinical algorithms, as well as specific ones, over the past three years. The Agency for Health Care Policy and Research and the American Medical Association have collected clinical guidelines, and the Agency is supporting establishment of an internet-based guideline clearing house. These sources can be contacted by e-mail, and the addresses are posted on the following web sites: "http://www.ahcpr.gov" and "http://www.ama-assn.org." In addition, a single fairly comprehensive collection of more than 1,100 guideline summaries and 400 full-text guidelines has now been published on internet-linked CD-ROM by Faulkner and Gray (Faulkner and Gray's 1997 Practice Guidelines CD-ROM).

The following subsections introduce two aspects of guideline writing and revision: a systematic approach for writing guidelines, and the role of the guideline tender.

Using a Systematic Approach to Writing Guidelines Even if you don't have to write the guideline from scratch, in order to critique one effectively, you should have some practice using a critical, systematic approach to writing one. If the guideline is a new one, we strongly recommend first documenting the clinician's management logic by constructing a clinical algorithm. For most clinicians, a few hours practice using the rules in the Society for Medical Decision Making's proposed clinical algorithm standards should be sufficient for drafting an initial clinical logic map.[2] Clinicians less experienced in drawing algorithms can then benefit considerably from working with an experienced nonclinician algorithm writer. You will find exercises on constructing clinical algorithm maps (both from scratch and from a text version of clinical management) and on converting text to flow chart, or algorithmization,[3] at the back of this chapter.

Let us assume, then, that you now have some skill in drawing a clinical algorithm and that the guideline you are proposing to use is the American Academy of Pediatrics asthma management guideline. The next step would be to systematically critique the guideline. One approach to doing such a critique can be found in exercise 5 at the back of this chapter. There are other examples given for you to work out if you wish.

Appointing a Guideline Tender   To our knowledge, Gordon Moore, the well-known medical education innovator, first coined the term "guideline tender." His concept was that just as a shepherd tends his or her sheep, an algorithm tender would care for and nurture his or her algorithms. Depending on the organizational setting, the tender might be the person who chooses a guideline, writes it from scratch, edits it, or monitors its implementation. Editing a guideline seed, as anyone who has tried it knows, is hard work. However, the work does not end with a final draft or "penultimate draft" (step 6). In practice, there is no absolute final draft, because a guideline should be revised every six months to two years. No guideline is complete unless it not only is dated but also carries a renewal date. Even this commitment to continuous revision is not enough. Ideally, there should be a mechanism for providing the person responsible for the update with an ongoing review of the literature, so that if a striking new finding changes patient management significantly, the guideline could be updated at any time.

This is not to say that guidelines cannot be implemented without a tender; they can. In some settings, the tender will not even be very involved with implementation. However, from the quality perspective, a clinician who has a commitment to caring for the central clinical problem is the best-qualified person to update the guideline effectively. A guideline tender, then, is the person or persons who worry about all aspects of guideline construction and revision.

Step 2. Marshal the Evidence

Whether or not this step comes first, the basic procedures are the same. Two sorts of literature review must be done by an experienced clinician aiming to draft a guideline. First, he or she should examine several textbook or review article descriptions of managing the clinical problem. Even an experienced clinician will want to do this in order to assure him- or herself that his or her knowledge of management is complete and to clarify possible disparities between his or her approach and the clinical approach described in the literature. Second, all recent research relevant to clinical management should be reviewed and graded as to quality of evidence. A detailed discussion of these procedures is beyond the scope of this book, but chapter 3 deals in depth with the relationship between evidence and guideline recommendations.

Step 3. Perform Consensus Processing

How does one determine recommendations for practice when there is no evidence or no quality evidence available, or when the evidence is conflicting? Proponents of evidence-based clinical guidelines tend to be sharply critical of consensus procedures. However, much of practice consists of decisions that are considered accepted, rational practice, but are not based on evidence. To give one of a myriad of examples, treatment of allergic contact dermatitis, such as poison ivy, commonly involves deciding whether the episode is the patient's first or is a repeat. Severe first episodes might be treated with a short course of high-dose steroids that are discontinued without tapering, but steroids are usually reserved for patients with repeat episodes and are used for periods of a week or more with tapering. The rationale for the use of longer-term steroids with tapering in repeat episodes is that repeat episodes last several weeks rather than a matter of days and that steroids reduce inflammation rapidly, but might cause rebound rash if not tapered over time.

To our knowledge, no double-blind controlled study has shown that steroids are effective, what their complication rate is, or what the rebound rate is in either first or subsequent episodes of poison ivy. We feel strongly, however, that it is essential to teach and practice clinical management of allergic contact dermatitis in a consistent manner, one buttressed by pathophysiological reasoning and guided by the principle of reducing harm, whether or not the evidence is available. The alternative would be that in every case of first episode or repeat severe allergic contact dermatitis, the physician might or might not decide to use steroids and the result might be many days of suffering for patients whose rash, if treated, would have resolved rapidly. Of course, if the treatment effect is in serious doubt, we would prefer that a proper effectiveness trial be performed.

Even Don Berwick, who is a strong supporter of clinical guidelines, when asked at one of the original Harvard Community Health Plan clinical guideline development workshops to define clinical guideline validity, answered, "I suppose that a valid clinical algorithm would be one for which each of the decisions is supported by a decision analysis." Asked whether all clinical algorithms would reach this level of validity, he answered, "Well, it seems unlikely—at least in my lifetime." Less favorably inclined critics of consensus have pointed out that tyro as well as expert clinicians have been shown to make decisions that frequently lack sufficient evidence. Even when shown the evidence, consensus groups do not always reach a consensus consistent with the evidence.

We agree with all these criticisms. We also agree that it is useful to strive toward obtaining evidence to support the decisions in a clinical guideline. However, a large part of clinical medicine is not currently supported by any evidence. This does not mean we should stop attempting to collect the evidence. But it also does not mean that when there is no available evidence we should stop making decisions about patients. If we did, much of medical practice would cease instantly. Our approach is to do the following:

1. Base as much of the algorithm map seed as possible on evidence.
2. Make the evidence available to the consensus group in easily digestible form.
3. Use structured, tested consensus procedures such as nominal group process[4, 5] and a Delphi[6, 7] process to reach consensus efficiently on the map and on the clinical guideline (both the nominal group process and the Delphi process are described in the last section of this chapter).

Step 4. Write the First Revision of the Algorithm Seed

To revise the seed, two or three members of the consensus group should take responsibility for editing. Choosing the editors depends on somewhat different factors in different settings, but three factors that almost always should be taken into account are personal initiative, the structure of the institution's clinical guideline program, and the clinical guideline topic.

I remember working with a pneumonia clinical guideline consensus group that included a very quiet woman who was the local pulmonologist. When I asked for volunteers, to my surprise she immediately raised her hand. The only other volunteer was a primary care physician who had been kibitzing so frequently that I was sure he was hardly taking the consensus process seriously. I realized, however, that the advantages in choosing these two were that I would have a local subject expert who was a potential user and a clinician who was very familiar with the clinical problem. We attached a clinical guidelines expert to these two unlikely partners, and in two days they produced one of the best second drafts I have seen.

No matter what considerations are employed to determine the editors, a significant improvement in the next draft depends on subject input and technical input. Increasingly, clinical guideline users are realizing that technical input, such as formatting, logic checking, and using appropriate computerized graphics, is essential for producing a high-quality clinical guideline revision. In its new systemwide clinical guideline program, the Veterans Health Administration has set aside special support for this sort of technical critiquing of their new clinical guidelines.

To process the results of any sort of consensus program effectively, the editors must proceed systematically. We use the following editing rules for the nominal group process:

- If the consensus comment has majority support from the group, it should be retained in the new draft, unless the editors disagree(!). In the latter case, they may exercise editorial power and choose to not put the comment into the revision. However, they must then make explicit this choice and its rationale when they return the clinical guideline to the consensus group for review.
- If the consensus comment does not have majority support, then the reverse of the above procedure is used. Again, the editors may exercise their editorial license to put into the revised draft a weakly supported recommendation, so long as the change is clearly presented to the consensus group, which may then overrule them.

These two rules on the one hand enable the editors, who after all are most familiar with the clinical guideline draft, to have the strongest effect on it. On the other hand, final changes remain the prerogative of the entire consensus group.

- If at all possible, editing should be done on an electronic version of the draft, using Macflow, Winflow, or other software specially designed to construct flowcharts. These rules are adapted from those used to produce revised Delphi drafts. In the Delphi process, editing drafts is an integral part of the process. However, there is usually one editor who controls editing absolutely and is required to feed back all changes to the group, whether or not he or she has used them in the revision.

Step 5. Repeat Iterations of Steps 3 and 4

How many times should the consensus group process the seed guideline? In the initial methodological work on Delphi process, it was shown that comments diminished considerably after the first round and were minimal after the second round. R. H. Brooke, the well-known health services research expert, made similar observations on the medical Delphi processes that he performed. Keeping these observations in mind, we use the process shown in table 2-1 to produce a final draft. The total time required to produce a guideline seed using this method comes to about six weeks.

TABLE 2-1. Process for Producing a Guideline Seed

Process Step	Time Required*	Who
1. Produce seed 1.1 Write seed 1.2 Review literature	c. 1 month	Experienced clinician + guideline expert (ECGE) + assistant to review literature
2. NGP on seed	2 hours	Guideline expert
3. Draft #1	3 days	ECGE
4. NGP #2 on Draft #1	1.5 hours	Guideline expert
5. Draft #2	2 days	ECGE
6. Optional Delphi: let group decide	1 week	ECGE

*Times are maximum estimates, except for literature review time, which depends on how much assistance is available.

Many variations on this guideline development process are possible. However, they invariably will involve generating a seed and multiple drafts. Using this process, we were able to produce advanced drafts of the World Health Organization's long and complex Global Program on AIDS Guidelines for HIV/AIDS Management in Children in about one month.[8] Although we started with an advanced seed (the Global Program on AIDS Guidelines for HIV/AIDS Management in Adults), starting from scratch would only have added another month.[9]

Step 6. Write the Penultimate Draft

The penultimate draft of almost all the guidelines we have worked on was written after not more than three rounds of consensus processing. This draft should be as carefully edited for technical and graphical errors as for content errors; it should be dated; and it should bear the names of the individuals working in its consensus group. Practical questions at this point are, "Who should 'sign off' on the draft?"; "What should 'signing off' entail?"; and "Is this the draft that gets implemented?"

Who Should Sign Off on the Draft? Little has been written as yet about "signing off" or gaining official approval of a guideline, but we feel that this seemingly straightforward process is the cause of most of the delay in guideline development.

At the local level, when the guidelines have been either developed in-house or locally tailored, "signing off" involves making sure to gain the approval of anyone who has not been directly involved with developing the guideline but will be involved in its implementation. For example, before implementing a breast biopsy guideline at a large health maintenance organization, approval was also sought from the chief physicians of the surgery, radiology, and pathology services, even though members of these departments participated in developing the guideline and a general surgeon was the guideline tender.

In-house sign-off might take several weeks or even months, but it is a necessary implementation step. However, formal approval of a guideline that is being developed at a higher level, for example, by a national specialty organization or by the Agency for Health Care Policy and Research, might get bogged down for many months, or even years, in a morass of political or scientific reservations.

Consider the following example of political problems. The World Health Organization started developing its guidelines for Management of HIV/AIDS in Children in March 1990 with an efficient four-day nominal group process–based consensus conference that was aimed at modifying the already completed draft of the adult guidelines. An initial draft was complete within a month. Final approval of all guideline committee members was obtained within two months, and a carefully edited version was ready by September 1990—yet the guidelines were published in December 1994! Another example is the American Academy of Pediatrics' Hyperbilirubinemia in the Normal Newborn Practice Parameter, which took close to two years to finish, even though an advanced draft was ready within six months of beginning the project.

Much of the the World Health Organization delay was due to internal inefficiency caused by large organization slowness, internal reorganizations, redundancy of internal approvals, and an inefficient publishing mechanism. However, significant delays were also caused by delaying final approval until initial buy-in by some countries was secured. Most of the hyperbilirubinemia delay, however, was caused by repeated revisions by neonatologists and primary care pediatricians.

Another example is the long gestation time of the American Academy of Pediatrics Otitis Media Practice Parameter, brought about by the need to gain approval from other professional societies. Perhaps the most extreme example is the Agency for Health Care Policy and Research backing away from the area of developing guidelines, in part because the Academy of Orthopedic Surgeons disagreed with the recommendation of chiropractic as an alternative low back pain therapy and threatened to bring legal action if the guideline was published.

What Should Signing Off Entail? At present, there is no procedure for avoiding these pitfalls and shortening these disturbing delays. However, several actions should be taken in the long run to make the approval process more efficient and effective. These actions include the following:

1. Research on the exact nature of the delays that would aid in pre-
    venting them
2. Policymakers and managers realizing that clinical guidelines are
    not written in stone and, therefore, do not imply unchangeable
    legal documents that mandate practice be done only in one way
3. When approval is requested from an individual, making clear at
    the outset that it relates mainly to scientific content and, if
    there are other considerations, asking the person approving to
    identify them and the guideline tender to process these prob-
    lems separately

Is This the Draft That Gets Implemented? The answer is yes—and
no. The "signed-off" penultimate draft is ready to be processed for
implementation, but one should never assume that the penultimate draft
will be implemented without further processing. The history of clinical
practice guidelines, from the first clinical algorithm systems in the 1960s
to the present, is strewn with stories of unsuccessful implementation.
Many of them have involved the assumption that a well-researched,
clearly considered, and carefully drawn guideline can be plugged in and
turned on like a toaster. However, clinical practice guidelines are not
toasters. They are, as we will explain in detail in chapter 6, complex decision guides that enable a team of clinicians and administrators to design
an action plan, a system that enables the guideline decisions to be
effected in the real world of providers and patients.

Just as a clinical algorithm is the logic engine that drives a clinical
practice guideline, the clinical practice guideline is the conceptual blue-
print for the design of the clinical practice guidelines system. This system consists of four components:

1. The patient and his or her family
2. The clinical team
3. The nonclinical infrastrucuture of care
4. Specific clinical practice guidelines aimed at caring for the
    patient's problem

These four components are connected functionally by two linked
processes—the guideline development cycle and the guideline implementation cycle—described in the introduction as "The Guidelines Bi-
cycle" (see figure FM-1). The three-step guideline development cycle is
linked to the six-step implementation cycle at the implementation step,
which is common to both cycles. Only when this system has been carefully constructed should one attempt to "ride the bicycle"—that is, to
operationalize a clinical practice guideline. Guideline design and development was step 2 in the guideline development cycle. Chapter 3 offers

an in-depth discussion of how to build evidence into guidelines. For a discussion of the next step in the guideline development cycle, dissemination and learning, see chapter 4.

CRITIQUING AND MODIFYING AN EXISTING GUIDELINE

Notice that the six steps of the clinical practice guideline development process described above can be used not only to develop a guideline, but also to critique and modify an existing one. Key techniques for either developing a new guideline or modifying an existing one are those for linking evidence to the guideline and for reaching a consensus efficiently. Chapter 3 deals at length with evidence linking. Let us now consider the two major consensus-processing techniques in detail.

Nominal Group Process

The nominal group process was first introduced to the medical field in 1971, and I learned it in 1972 from a social scientist who had learned it directly from its inventors.[10] As fellows at the Office of Medical Education Research and Development at Michigan State University, my colleagues and I used it to define the problems of our fellowship program. I have since initiated or participated in hundreds of nominal group processes on many different topics, but they all have had the same general purpose: to define problems in a specific area.

Personal Examples of Nominal Group Process Participation   The longest and perhaps most significant nominal group process that I led was in 1988 with Joe Pliskin, the medical decision-making expert, and Yair Shapiro, professor of physiology and then medical director of the Soroka University Hospital, and aimed at "defining the problems of the Soroka University Hospital." It took three Friday mornings (about nine hours!) to produce a prioritized list of 60 problems that were then broken up into eight problem groups. The plan for each problem group was developed by a three-person team.

In contrast, most of the nominal group processes I have done are aimed at critiquing a guideline and have produced a corrected guideline draft. The most difficult nominal group process I have ever done was the one with Wilfred Lorenz, expert in clinical decision making and clinical trials, in January 1997, that enabled a group of 14 general surgeons from six countries to critique a guideline for management of surgical sepsis.

Steps in the Nominal Group Process Here are some tips on leading a nominal group process. They are based on following the steps outlined in table 2-2.

First, distribute the seed algorithm and its supporting literature. You may mail relevant clinical literature to participants before the session. In many cases the participants will not have read it before the meeting, so it is almost always useful to give them a few minutes to review the literature before the work begins, and then to summarize it. Then, explain that this is a structured group process (in contrast to discussion in the British Parliament or Israeli Knesset, which have rules but frequently deteriorate into shouting matches and are inefficient). You, the group leader, must explain the rules clearly and stick to them. Tell the group to think of the nominal group process as a game. Postpone discussion of the process itself for the end, even if the group is doing this for the first time. Explain that it will learn more by commenting after it has experienced the process.

Second, have the participants review the seed and note specific comments. I jump-start the process by setting aside some time (usually between 7 and 15 minutes, depending on the material to be reviewed) to review the guideline and any other materials, and write down any and all comments. Ask the participants to try to phrase them as suggestions for change and to remember that at this point there will be no talking or discussion. Then, have the participants begin. Use a stopwatch. Warn the group when time is almost up. You can add a few minutes if people haven't finished, but don't be too generous. Continue at a crisp pace.

Third, have the participants state comments—the leader will record them. When time for review is up, announce to the group, "We're going to collect comments in the following way: we will go around the room and each of you will read aloud all your comments that have not been stated. I will record and number all comments on the flip chart. Still there will be no discussion, but you can ask for a clarification if it is not clear to you whether a comment on the chart is the same as the one you have written."

TABLE 2-2. Steps in the Nominal Group Process

- Distribute "Seed algorithm" and supporting literature
- Participants review seed, and note specific comments
- Participants state comments, recorded by leader
- Comments are "collapsed"
- Vote
- Participants discuss
- Seed reconstructed, including majority opinion
- Further processing until consensus is reached

Reprinted, with permission, from *Designing Care Coursebook,* published by the Institute for Healthcare Improvement, Boston, © 1991–1996.

Another way to do this is to let each participant give only one comment at a time, going around the room several times until there are no more comments left. Either method works, but the first one is probably a bit faster, and the second is probably a bit more fair. A frequent comment is that using the whole list method, the last people get tired of waiting their turn and might be able to contribute only a few comments. I have not found this to be a problem.

Fourth, collapse comments that seem similar. This will help make efficient the process of prioritization, because the vote will consider groups of comments rather than each individual comment. Note comment groups on the flip chart by drawing a line through the number of the comment to be grouped without erasing its comment text, and then writing that number next to the first comment of the group. As people shout out suggestions for grouping problems, the list will be modified to show a group of comment numbers next to each major comment and many other "moved" comments that have their numbers crossed out but have not been erased.

Fifth, vote. Ask, "How are we going to prioritize this list?" Read out every comment in a problem group and allow each participant to vote for or against each group. Ask, "So, what is the maximum number of votes in favor of any comment?" It usually takes the group a few minutes to realize that it equals the number of participants (of course)! "And," I ask slyly, "what is the minimum number of votes in favor of any comment?" They are slower in realizing that the minimum number is zero, since the person who proposed a comment might have decided during the discussion to vote against it. When we finish voting, each comment, or group of collapsed comments, has a colored number near the beginning that tells how many voted in favor.

Part of this step is determining who the editors are going to be. After two or three editors have been appointed, explain the editing rules (discussed earlier in this chapter):

- If the comment has more than half of the votes, it must be retained in the new draft, unless the editors disagree. If the latter is the case, the editors can drop the comment, providing they explain what they have done when they present the new draft to the group.
- The converse also holds. If the editors want to retain a comment that has earned less than half of the votes, they may do so, provided they present the change and their explanation.

Sixth, discuss. Usually there is very little discussion. The process of thinking through whether someone else's comments are the same as yours and then presenting your own has usually replaced most of the discussion. However, discussion can elicit useful or even important suggestions for modifying the guideline overall. For example, during the discussion phase of a nominal group process on pneumonia management, a participant suggested switching the position of an algorithm branch that saved the editors a significant amount of time.

Delphi Process

My first Delphi attempted to achieve consensus on criteria for management of pneumonia in children. Working from the first description of Delphi in the *New England Journal of Medicine* and from a description by a colleague who had done many of them, I began by soliciting cooperation from all the clinicians who I thought would be directly involved with gathering the data or using the results of the audit.

The Delphi process, first described by social scientist N. C. Dalkey in 1969, feels quite different from nominal group process.[11] Its purpose is to derive an estimate from a knowledgeable group or to reach group consensus on a draft. Again, the most useful, practical hint is to follow the steps listed in table 2-3. Here are a few comments on those steps:

First, distribute the "seed algorithm" and its supporting literature. Distribute this by mail, fax, or e-mail. The participants will never meet—this eliminates group interaction, for better or worse, but increases the Delphi leader's power considerably.

Second, request comments to be returned by a firm deadline set in a short amount of time (within one month). Make it clear to participants when enlisting them that failure to meet deadlines will result in their being dropped from the process.

Third, collate the comments. Start with the longest list of comments. Read the first comment and then check to see how many of the other participants listed it. Tally the "votes" for each comment, record the number next to the comment, and then mark the comment "used up." When all the comments on the longest list have been voted

---

TABLE 2-3. Steps in the Delphi Process

- Distribute "seed algorithm" and supporting literature
- Request specific comments to be returned by firm deadline
- Collage the comments
- Reconstruct the seed, including majority opinion
- Send collated comments, and revised algorithm, back to group for further comments (return to step 2) until consensus

Reprinted, with permission, from *Designing Care Coursebook,* published by the Institute for Healthcare Improvement, Boston, © 1991–1996.

for, move to the next longest list and tally the votes for all the unused comments. Repeat this process until there are no unused comments on any list. All the lists together will constitute a prioritized list of comments, each of which either has been crossed out or has a number of votes.

Fourth, reconstruct the seed—edit the draft. Use the same rules used in editing the nominal group process draft. In a classic Delphi, the draft with all corrections is returned to the participants for comment, and then this process is repeated until there are no more comments. I remember a classical Delphi on routine preventive practices in adults that was still going on after two years!

Fifth, send the collated comments and revised algorithm back to the group for further comments. When given the chance to see others' comments, participants cannot seem to refrain from commenting just one more time. Since, however, comments almost always diminish sharply after round two, we arbitrarily stop the Delphi after two rounds.

QUESTIONS FOR STUDY

1. What is the situation in which it is pointless to attempt writing a clinical practice guideline?
2. What are three indications for developing a clinical practice guideline?
3. What are three essential elements of a quality clinical practice guideline?
4. What are six commonly followed stages in developing a clinical practice guideline?
5. What are two essential steps in critiquing a clinical practice guideline?
6. What are three essential procedures for reviewing the literature?
7. What are two structured group processes for reaching a consensus?
8. Are nominal group process and Delphi mutually exclusive techniques?
9. What sort of expertise and group interest should be represented in the guideline editing group? How many editors should there be?
10. What is the basic rule for editing a clinical practice guideline consensus draft?
11. What is a guideline tender?
12. What are two necessary sorts of "signing off"?
13. Is the penultimate draft the draft implementation plan?

The answers to these questions can be found in Appendix B.

PROBLEMS AND EXERCISES

Exercise 1. How to Draw an Algorithm Map

The state of Massachusetts is strongly considering enabling new drivers to learn skills using algorithms. On a separate sheet of paper, draw your own algorithm flowchart for teaching someone to drive through an intersection governed by a traffic light, without referring to Feinstein's attempt in chapter 1. Make use of the standard clinical algorithm symbols for drawing clinical algorithm flowcharts.[12]

Standard Symbols:

Clinical State or Problem Definition

Diagnostic Decision

Do (Action) Box

Standard Numbering
and Annotating

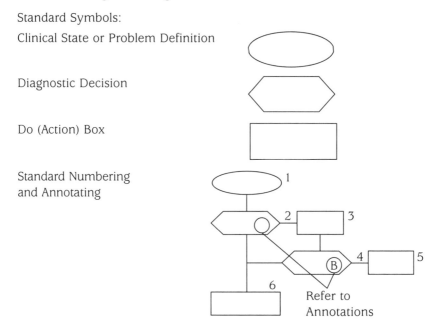

Number from top to bottom, but number right-hand branches before continuing down the trunk. This is an arbitrary but consistent system. Its main purpose is to facilitate referring to decision boxes.

Exercise 2. How to Draw a Clinical Algorithm Map

Now that you have practiced drawing an algorithm map for a nonclinical problem, try your hand at a clinical problem. Any clinical problem you work with is fine, but we will use pharyngitis, a clinical problem that many clinicians are familiar with, as an example.

On a separate sheet of paper, draw a clinical algorithm for a patient older than five years who presents with a sore throat and an erythematous pharynx. Follow the steps in table 2-4, "How to Write a Clinical Algorithm."

TABLE 2-4. How to Write a Clinical Algorithm

Define the problem	Users Patient population Resources
Differential diagnosis	List all causes Review pathophysiology
Sequencing of boxes	Clinical state box Most urgent Most common Rare causes in annotations
Specify therapy	Drugs and dosages Monitor treatment
Specify end points	Functional status Referral Discharge
Annotations	Clarify rationale Explain controversy Expand information in box Review less essential details omitted from algorithm

Reprinted, with permission, from *Designing Care Coursebook,* published by the Institute for Healthcare Improvement, Boston, © 1991–1996.

Exercise 3. Algorithmization

On a separate sheet of paper, convert the following clinical list format coronary heart disease guidelines to a flowchart:

Protocol for the Management of Coronary Heart Disease: List Format (further information is contained in the Coronary Heart Disease Health of the National Task Group Report published by East Riding Health Authority, UK, May 1994).

Patients with chest pain, suspicion of unstable angina (that is, recent onset of chest pain; deteriorating pattern of chest pain; pain occurring at rest or at night):

- Consider referral to the chest pain clinic
- Commence treatment with aspirin (75–300 mg) and a beta blocker
- Closely monitor symptoms and treatment
- Review early—consider cardiological assessment

Patients with suspected myocardial infarct (that is, suggestive cardiac pain lasting longer than 15 minutes, particularly if at rest or accompanied by dyspnoea, sweating, or nausea):

- If cannot attend within 10 minutes, call emergency ambulance— refer to hospital
- Give aspirin, 300 mg as single dose (ideally chewed); only contraindication is definite aspirin allergy
- Give analgesia (opoid) if required; use with antimetic—use IV route if possible

Patients with previous myocardial infarct:

- All patients should receive long-term aspirin treatment, 75–300 mg a day
- All patients should receive long-term beta blockade unless contraindicated
- Consider referral for cardiological assessment, stress testing, or further investigation
- Check lipid status and consider diet or drug therapy; where serum cholesterol is >5.5 mmol/L, try a cholesterol-lowering diet for six months; retest—if total cholesterol is >5.5 mmol/L, try a cholesterol-lowering drug

Patients with established (stable) coronary disease:

- Consider cardiological assessment
- All patients should receive long-term aspirin treatment, 75–300 mg a day
- Consider beta blockade where possible

Exercise 4. Algorithmization—Nonclinical

On a separate sheet of paper, convert the following text to an algorithm:

Leprosy management: Leviticus, 13: 3–4.

EXHIBIT 2-1. Leprosy Algorithm

1010	And the priest shall look on the plague in the skin of the flesh; and
1011	If the hair of the plague be turned white, and the appearance of the plague be deeper than the skin of his flesh, Then it is the plague of leprosy (tzara'at). And
1012	If the bright spot be white in the skin of his flesh, and the appearance thereof be not deeper than the skin, and hair thereof be not turned white, Then the priest shall shut him up that hath the plague 7 days.

Leviticus 13: 3–4, c. 1230 BC; programmed in Hebrew, translated by J. H. Hertz, 1972.

Exercise 5. Critiquing a Clinical Practice Guideline

On a separate sheet of paper, critique the East Riding Health Authority coronary heart disease guideline from exercise 3 using the enclosed Appraisal Instrument for Clinical Guidelines. The Instrument has been followed, using the coronary heart disease guideline as the one being critiqued.

Solutions to these problems and exercises can be found in Appendix B.

EXHIBIT 2-2. Appraisal Instrument for Clinical Guidelines

	Yes	No	Not sure	Not applicable	Notes
Dimension 1: Rigour of Development					
Responsibility for guideline development					
1. Is the agency responsible for the development of the guidelines clearly identified?					
2. Was external funding or other support received for developing the guideline?					
3. If external funding or support was received, is there evidence that the potential biases of the funding body(ies) were taken into account?					
Guideline development group					
4. Is there a description of the individuals (e.g., professionals, interest groups—including patients) who were involved in the guidelines development group?					
5. If so, did the group contain representatives of all key disciplines?					
Identification and interpretation of evidence					
6. Is there a description of the sources of information used to select the evidence on which the recommendations are based?					
7. If so, are the sources of information adequate?					
8. Is there a description of the method(s) used to interpret and assess the strength of the evidence?					
9. If so, is (are) the method(s) for rating the evidence satisfactory?					

EXHIBIT 2-2. (Continued)

	Yes	No	Not sure	Not applicable	Notes
Dimension 1: Rigour of Development					
Formulation of recommendations					
10. Is there a description of the methods used to formulate the recommendations?					
11. If so, are the methods satisfactory?					
12. Is there an indication of how the views of interested parties not on the panel were taken into account?					
13. Is there an explicit link between the major recommendations and the level of supporting evidence?					
Peer review					
14. Were the guidelines independently reviewed prior to their publication/ release?					
15. If so, is explicit information given about methods and how comments were addressed?					
16. Were the guidelines piloted?					
17. If the guidelines were piloted, is explicit information given about the methods used and the results adopted?					
Updating					
18. Is there a mention of a date for reviewing or updating the guidelines?					
19. Is the body responsible for the reviewing and updating clearly identified?					

(Continued on next page)

EXHIBIT 2-2. (Continued)

	Yes	No	Not sure	Not applicable	Notes
Dimension 1: Rigour of Development *Overall assessment of development process*					
20. Overall, have the potential biases of guideline development been adequately dealt with?					
Dimension 2: Context and Content *Objectives*					
21. Are the reasons for developing the guidelines clearly stated?					
22. Are the objectives of the guidelines clearly defined?					
Context					
23. Is there a satisfactory description of the patients to which the guidelines are meant to apply?					
24. Is there a description of the circumstances (clinical or non clinical) in which exceptions might be made in using the guidelines?					
25. Is there an explicit statement of how patients' preferences should be taken into account in applying the guidelines?					
Clarity					
26. Do the guidelines describe the condition to be detected, treated, or prevented in unambiguous terms?					
27. Are the different possible options for management of the condition clearly stated in the guidelines?					
28. Are the recommendations clearly presented?					

EXHIBIT 2-2. (Continued)

	Yes	No	Not sure	Not applicable	Notes
Dimension 2: Context and Content					
Likely costs and benefits					
29. Is there an adequate description of the health benefits that are likely to be gained from the recommended management?					
30. Is there an adequate description of the potential harms or risks that may occur as a result of the recommended management?					
31. Is there an estimate of the costs or expenditures likely to incur from the recommended management?					
32. Are the recommendations supported by the estimated benefits, harms, and costs of the intervention?					
Dimension 3: Application					
Guideline dissemination & implementation					
33. Does the guideline document suggest possible methods for dissemination and implementation?					
Monitoring of guidelines/clinical audit					
34. Does the guideline document specify criteria for monitoring compliance?					
35. Does the guideline document identify clear standards or targets?					
36. Does the guideline document define measurable outcomes that can be monitored?					
National guidelines only					
37. Does the guideline document identify key elements which need to be considered by local guideline groups?					

Reprinted, with permission, from Cluzeau F., Littlejohns P., Grimshaw J., Feder G., Appraisal Instrument for Clinical Guidelines. Version 1, published by St. George's Hospital Medical School, London, May 1997.

References and Notes

1. C. Z. Margolis, S. Warshawsky, L. Goldman, O. Dagan, D. Wirtschafter, and J. S. Pliskin, "Computerized Algorithms and Pediatricians' Management of Common Problems in a Community Clinic," *Acad. Med.* 67 (1992): 282.

2. Society for Medical Decision Making Committee on Standardization of Clinical Algorithms, "Proposal for Clinical Algorithm Standards," *Med. Dec. Making* 12, no. 2 (1992):149–54.

3. Algorithmization: This awkward, almost unpronounceable term refers to converting a text or list format algorithm to a flowchart format. It is of course a misnomer, since the original text or list format is no less a description of an algorithm than is the flowchart.

4. A. Donabedian, *The Criteria and Standards of Quality* (Ann Arbor, MI: Health Administration Press, 1982).

5. A. Fink, et al., "Consensus Methods: Characteristics and Guidelines for Use," *Am. J. Public Health* 74 (1984): 979–83.

6. N. C. Dalkey, *The Delphi Method: An Experimental Study of Group Opinion* (Santa Monica, CA: The Rand Corporation, 1969).

7. A. Donabedian, *The Delphi Technique* (Santa Monica, CA: The Rand Corporation, 1969), pp. 154–9.

8. WHO Guidelines for Children, "Global Program on AIDS Guidelines for Management of HIV/AIDS in Children," World Health Organization, Geneva, 1991.

9. WHO Guidelines for Adults. "Global Program on AIDS Guidelines for Management of HIV/AIDS in Adults," World Health Organization, Geneva, 1991.

10. A. Delbecq and A Van de Ven, "A Group Process Model for Problem Identification and Program Planning," *J. Appl. Behav. Sci.* 7 (1971): 467–92.

11. Dalkey, *Delphi Method.*

12. Society, "Clinical Algorithm Standards."

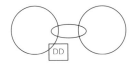

3

Building in the Evidence

Robert H. Fletcher, MD, MSc

C linical guidelines should be based on the best available evidence. That is easy to say but far more difficult to put into practice. For example, consider the panel members who are to prepare the guideline. They are chosen for the expertise they can bring to bear on the work, and they are likely to be confident that they know their task. But when they begin to examine the scientific evidence, they might find that they are having difficulty agreeing. They might attribute this to a few difficult members—and they might be right. But the difficulties also could have arisen because they, and the organizing body that charged the panel, have not first grappled with several questions that are even more fundamental to the work than the evidence itself. If these questions are not dealt with clearly, early in the guidelines process, they will come back to haunt the panel in innumerable ways. What might appear to be personal disagreements; self-interest on the part of one or another special interest group; or arguments about the fine points of study design, measurement, and analyses might be related to failure to confront and resolve these issues. If so, the authority and usefulness of the resulting guideline will be weakened.

This chapter explores the scientific underpinnings of guidelines, how the science is judged, and how it is included when writing guidelines. The chapter is divided into eight key questions that panel members should address before completing the work of writing guidelines.

WHO IS QUALIFIED TO JUDGE THE EVIDENCE?

Is it only "experts" who are highly specialized in the clinical content area: urologists for prostate problems, psychiatrists for depression, and so on? Or is there a place for other stakeholders with different experiences and

47

perspectives, such as primary care physicians, decision analysts, or even patients and their families?

Guideline writing has traditionally been the purview of clinicians who are highly specialized in the clinical condition being considered. Often the project is sponsored by their specialty society. Thus, the American Heart Association produces a guideline on the prevention of endocarditis, the American Thoracic Society on asthma, the American Cancer Society on cancers, and so on.

Certainly, this approach has many strengths. These specialists are likely to have extensive experience in the care of patients with the condition in question. They are likely to be familiar with published research and might have been authors of many of the relevant studies. They often find it easy to agree on what should be recommended, since they and their colleagues have discussed the issues many times and have long since agreed among themselves about what should be done, believing that all that remains is to write down their views for the rest of the world.

Ramifications of Using a Purely Specialty Panel

There are a number of disadvantages to having guidelines written by a purely specialty panel. These include the following:

- The agreement might leave important questions, when viewed from other perspectives, unidentified and unexamined. Highly specialized physicians often see the issues very differently from other interested parties, not just because of their greater in-depth knowledge of the disease, but also because they see patients with diseases within a particular spectrum: patients who are already known to have the disease in which the physicians are specialized, have an unusual or severe manifestation of the disease, and are highly selected from the general population because of referral. This might not cover all aspects of the question addressed by the guideline. For example, if the guideline is about prevention, this kind of work takes place in the offices of primary care physicians.
- Experts might have a variety of biases or conflicts of interest that bear on their work. Even if they do not have a direct financial interest in a company selling one of the products being judged, they might earn their living by offering one of the very practices that are being considered in the guideline. For example, neurosurgeons and orthopedic surgeons are paid for doing back surgery and so might take a dim view of conservative management of back pain. In addition, specialists might be biased by "intellectual passion," an understandable, even desirable, belief in doing things the way they do them. They might also defer to

close friends and associates, especially if they look on the guide-line setting process as a pleasant diversion from their usual work, or if they are seeking elected office in the professional society that is sponsoring the guideline. What's more, they might mis-trust the scientific arguments, or even the integrity, of clinicians who offer alternatives to their kind of care—as, for example, when it comes to screening for colorectal cancer, some gastroen-terologists (who do colonoscopies) and radiologists (who do bar-ium enemas) mistrust each other.

- Expertise in a clinical specialty makes one no more or less qual-ified than other scholars in many of the other disciplines rele-vant to the guideline, because judging the scientific credibility of the research itself calls on skills in critical appraisal of research evidence.

All other participants can, of course, have the same array of biases and limitations. Therefore, there is an advantage to having a heteroge-neous panel.

Ramifications of Using a Heterogeneous Panel

A heterogeneous panel would represent the full range of disciplines that are relevant to the guidelines in question. These days, this would typically include the following:

- Subspecialty physicians
- Primary care physicians
- Nurses
- Nurse practitioners and physicians assistants
- Epidemiologists
- Behavior scientists
- Decision analysts
- Economists
- Ethicists
- Patients and families

What is achieved by such a mixture is not the absence of bias. Although conveners should attempt to select panel members with rela-tively open minds or at least transparent biases, each member of the panel will continue to have his or her own point of view, resulting from their individual experiences. What is achieved is a balancing of biases, especially if the decision-making process is open and each member of the panel feels that he or she has a voice. It is not the case that every-one's view is as good as everyone else's on every issue, but at least the panel should include a wide array of different kinds of expertise. What clinicians find self-evident, health policy analysts might find unfeasible (especially when cost or workforce are taken into account) and patients might find unacceptable. For example, although there is strong evidence that screening sigmoidoscopy prevents colorectal cancer, countries without ample resources for health care might not be able to choose this option and patients might find the prospect of the examination too daunting to accept advice to have it done.

Panels with balanced makeup have usually been convened by governmental organizations. Examples in the United States include the U.S. Preventive Services Task Force, a series of guidelines panels convened by the Agency for Health Care Policy and Research and the National Institutes of Health Consensus Development Conferences.

Unfortunately, such panels tend by their very nature to offend the usual experts, who feel ownership of the field. A notorious example is the reaction to a Consensus Development Panel convened by the National Institutes of Health to consider evidence concerning the effectiveness of screening mammography in women under 50 years in age. Their conclusion, that the evidence was not conclusive, was bitterly criticized by some radiologists, who are deeply invested in doing mammograms in these women.[1] In the United States, government panels have lost political favor in the wake of the partisan controversy that some guidelines have engendered. Government agencies have tended to withdraw from guideline-making activities and the work has reverted to specialty societies. Some view this as a step backward.[2]

Panels preparing guidelines at national or international levels have the resources and breadth of expertise necessary to review the evidence carefully and come to well-balanced conclusions—a process that commonly takes years to complete. An effort of this magnitude might not be possible for small groups of clinicians at the local level. Nevertheless, local physicians often are reluctant to accept guidelines by outsiders in their entirety because of either local pride or a genuine belief that the circumstances of their practice are different from practices in general. Tailoring national guidelines to the local practice environment, done by local clinicians, can both improve the guidelines' relevance and increase their credibility and, therefore, their use. Most often, the local panel will work with the evidence base developed by the national group, but apply somewhat different value judgments in making its recommendations. For example, my managed care organization, Harvard Pilgrim Health Care, reviews guidelines prepared by other expert groups and then prepares an extensive set of guidelines written by its own clinicians. The local recommendations are in the main similar to national guidelines for the same conditions.

The bottom line is this: Include subspecialists, to be sure, but also include members representing the full range of expertise that bears on the guideline, its implementation, and its consequences. What could be simpler in concept—and more difficult to accomplish? Guidelines can be very politically sensitive for all of the usual reasons—they deal with money, power, orthodoxy, and the emotions of people who have experienced disease or fear it.

WHAT KINDS OF QUESTIONS BEAR ON THE ADVICE BEING OFFERED?

Information on whether the interventions change the course of illness is important, certainly. But what about discomfort and inconvenience or severe injury and death caused by the intervention? What about cost—is it out of bounds?

Most clinical guidelines are about what clinicians or patients should do, that is, they are about interventions. So naturally, a central question is whether the interventions improve outcomes of care, traditionally measured as the five Ds: death, disease, disability, discomfort, and dissatisfaction. In modern times, another outcome of care is destitution, the sixth D. Other kinds of questions are also relevant, including the following:

- How much discomfort is engendered by the intervention? At stake is not only human suffering but also secondary effects on compliance. Patients might avoid experiences that cause them pain, nausea, fear, or embarrassment. They might tell their friends, who, when the intervention is recommended to them, refuse to participate. Clinicians tend to underestimate how difficult their procedures are, even "noninvasive" ones. One physician, while himself a patient, wrote of his experience with magnetic resonance imaging: "I was not prepared for the gargantuan monstrosity that confronted me, with its tiny mouth and its protruding tongue poised to lick me up and suck me inside. I lay down on the tongue, head first; I was strapped in and then covered with blankets because the room was chilly. Next, a cage was placed over my head. My slight claustrophobia was escalating. I was now fresh bait for the monster. Although skinny, I felt the scanner walls trapping my arms as I was sucked inside. . . . My mind began to race. If there is a fire, can I escape? With the cage against my shoulders, I felt my neck muscles tighten. . . . Then I felt an itch on my back that was growing in magnitude. I was ready to scream when the technician said, 'Okay, we're ready to take some pictures.'"[3]
- How convenient is the procedure? Does it involve days off work, travel over long distances, registering in an unfamiliar hospital,

forming personal relationships with strangers? Again, these affect both discomfort associated with health care and compliance.

- What risks result from the intervention? Nearly all interventions carry some possibility of serious complications or even death, either from the intervention itself or the downstream consequences of it (such as further diagnostic studies following a positive test, and medications and surgery for true and false positive results). Colonoscopy perforates the colon in about 1 to 3 patients per 1,000 colonoscopies. Coronary angiography can cause death, and some patients given penicillin experience anaphylaxis. At some level, the risk exceeds what might reasonably be undertaken to achieve the possible benefit. This level is usually well below the point at which risk and benefit are equally likely because patients tend to weigh harms caused by clinicians far more heavily than those caused by nature.

- What level of technical expertise is available to the patient? For example, the choice between open and laparoscopic cholecystectomy might be much less important than who does the procedure or where it is done. Often this information is not available. But there is a growing tendency in the United States to keep records on the outcomes of care for hospitals or even individual physicians, and to make these records publicly available. This follows a practice advocated by Dr. E. A. Codman in the early part of this century.[4]

- What are the costs of the interventions? Control of the rising cost of health care is a major public policy issue in nearly every developed country in the world. Yet cost is still not explicitly considered in most guideline processes. Most cost analyses take the "societal perspective," the theoretical cost to society as a whole, without regard to who pays or whether they are charged more or less than their own service costs. Unfortunately, the societal perspective has limited relevance to health care. "Society" does not pay bills—rather, an individual patient, insurer, or employer pays, or in prepaid health care the money is forgone by an individual physician or practice group. Moreover, those who must pay encounter charges, which might be a distorted representation of true costs because of accounting practices. So a central question is, "Charge to whom?"

- What is the cost-effectiveness of the intervention in relation to the alternatives? That is, what is the cost for each clinical effect, such as an added year of life? Cost-effectiveness might be very different from simple cost. For example, two screening tests for colorectal cancer—fecal occult blood testing and colonoscopy— have very different costs, about $5–10 and $400–1,000, respectively.[5] But their costs per year of life saved are about the same,

$18,000–20,000. Similarly, an expensive antibiotic for sepsis might cost less than an inexpensive one, when the expense of administration and treatment failures are taken into account.

The way in which cost has been included in the development of guidelines has been evolving in an irregular fashion through three phases:

1. Develop the guideline without consideration of cost.
2. Develop the guideline, then ask what the cost consequences would be.
3. Include consideration of cost and cost-effectiveness as an intrinsic part of the guideline process from the beginning.

We are just entering the third phase, with many guideline panels still firmly in the second or even the first phase. The way in which cost and cost-effectiveness are included, when they are included at all, ranges from formal cost-effectiveness analyses to reasoning based on qualitative information. In general, managed care organizations with responsibility for all aspects of care, including how it is paid for, are more likely to take cost into account when preparing guidelines than are professional organizations, which interpret their responsibilities mainly to promote quality of care and professional standards.

WHAT KIND OF SCIENTIFIC EVIDENCE IS ADMISSIBLE?

Large, randomized controlled trials, of course, are admissible, but are case reports, or expert opinion, or usual practice? Is a well-supported description of an intervention's mechanism of action essential or even sufficient without direct clinical studies?

Identifying the Validity of the Evidence

The evidence on which to base important decisions in the care of patients should meet high standards for validity. How is the best evidence identified?

Ensuring That All Interested Parties Can Examine the Evidence
It is common to insist that studies be published in peer-reviewed journals before they are considered. However, peer review and editing in even the most selective and prestigious journals, though they improve manuscripts,

do not guarantee that the published version is valid.[6] Therefore, guideline panel members cannot substitute the provenance of the article (its author, institution, journal) for their own careful review of the evidence.

The main issue is not, in any case, peer review. It is the opportunity for all interested parties to examine the full text of the article and to share views about the validity and meaning of the research. For this reason, some guideline panels consider unpublished manuscripts as long as they will be available to users of the guideline at the time it is released (so that they can examine the evidence base for themselves). An advantage is that including unpublished work makes up for the bias that published articles are more likely to have found statistically significant effects than are unpublished ones.[7] Abstracts of research generally are not used because they are not a full account of the works; also, it is not uncommon that the complete paper comes to different conclusions from the abstract or is even not published at all.

Choosing the Best Clinical Study Design   Often the best imaginable evidence, such as randomized controlled trials for the recommended versus alternative interventions, is not available, and one must settle for less. Figure 3-1 shows prototype designs for clinical research. Not all research fits into these molds, but they are the most common and the best understood ways of answering clinical questions. Note that the best kind of study design depends on the kind of question being asked, such as "How often does the condition occur?" or "What happens to people who develop the disease?"

Figure 3-2 shows the hierarchy of scientific strength for studies (provided they are done well) that attempt to determine whether something causes something else (treatment causes improvement, prevention causes people not to get the disease, or a risk factor causes disease).

In general, randomized controlled clinical trials of an intervention are the best way to determine whether that intervention, in and of itself, achieves its desired effects. The randomization removes the influence of other characteristics of the patient that might also affect the outcome. Observational studies, in which patients experience care as they normally would and the investigator observes interventions and outcomes, might be the best available evidence. But they have an inherent weakness: Other characteristics of the patient that might affect outcomes might be related to receiving the intervention and so be confused ("confounded") with the intervention being studied, misleading the reader. Much further down the hierarchy are reports of series of cases managed in a certain way. Their main limitation is that they include no strong point of comparison. Although their results can be compared to the outcomes of patients cared for in another way in another time and place, observed difference in interventions might not be the main reason for whatever differences in outcome are observed.

Characteristics of High-Quality Research This hierarchy applies only if the research itself (execution of the design, measurements, and analyses) is done well. Of the many important issues that might affect the validity of a study, beyond design, two stand out:

1. Whether the measurements (for example, measurement of whether the patient received the intervention, whether the

FIGURE 3-1. Research Designs and Questions

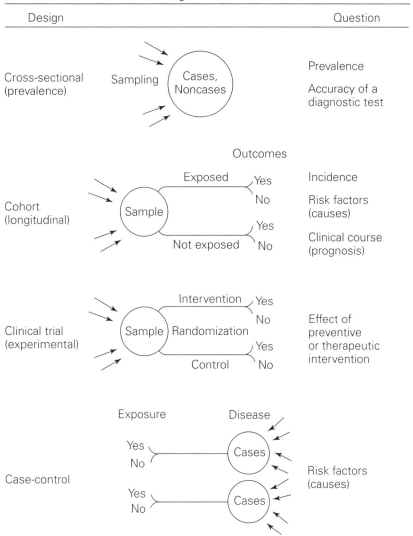

Design		Question
Cross-sectional (prevalence)	Sampling → Cases, Noncases	Prevalence Accuracy of a diagnostic test
Cohort (longitudinal)	Sample → Exposed (Yes/No), Not exposed (Yes/No) — Outcomes	Incidence Risk factors (causes) Clinical course (prognosis)
Clinical trial (experimental)	Sample → Randomization → Intervention (Yes/No), Control (Yes/No)	Effect of preventive or therapeutic intervention
Case-control	Exposure (Yes/No) → Cases; Exposure (Yes/No) → Cases — Disease	Risk factors (causes)

Reprinted, with permission, from R. H. Fletcher, S. W. Fletcher, and E. H. Wagner, *Clinical Epidemiology: The Essentials,* 3d ed. (Baltimore: Williams and Wilkins, 1996).

FIGURE 3-2. Hierarchy of Research Designs to Answer Whether an Intervention Is Effective

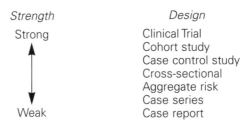

Strength	Design
Strong	Clinical Trial
↑	Cohort study
	Case control study
	Cross-sectional
↓	Aggregate risk
	Case series
Weak	Case report

Reprinted, with permission, from R. H. Fletcher, S. W. Fletcher, and E. H. Wagner, *Clinical Epidemiology: The Essentials,* 3d ed. (Baltimore: Williams and Wilkins, 1996).

patients receiving the intervention were otherwise similar to those who did not, or whether the outcome actually occurred) were unbiased—that is, whether they were unaffected by systematic error

2. Whether the contribution of chance to the findings is minimized or described (a relatively large number of patients must be included in order to arrive at a precise estimate of how large the true effect really is; stated in more technical terms, a large sample size is needed to arrive at a narrow confidence interval). Another approach to describing the role of chance, characterized by "p values," is to ask how strongly the study has ruled out the possibility that chance alone might have accounted for whatever differences (or lack of difference) were found. These two approaches are called "estimation" and "hypothesis testing," respectively.

Interpreting the Evidence

The language of clinical research, and the intricacies of judging individual studies, might not be familiar to many members of the panel who are otherwise well qualified in clinical care. What is the best method for interpreting the evidence so that it can be incorporated into the guideline? The following material describes three approaches.

Interpretation Based on Usual Practice Usual practice is worth mentioning, perhaps, but not as high-grade evidence in favor of a particular decision in a guideline. After all, if a guideline ends up recommending usual practice for its own sake, there is no reason to make the effort to prepare a guideline. The clinical community has already reached its goal! Moreover, there are plenty of examples where a course of action is soundly established by clinical research but is not part of usual practice.

An example is the strong, consistent, long-standing evidence that beta-blocking drugs reduce the mortality rate after acute myocardial infarction and a study showing that only 21 percent of eligible patients are receiving this treatment.[8]

Interpretation Based on the Mechanisms of Disease An appeal to the mechanisms of disease, apart from empirical studies of outcomes, occupies a special place in the culture of medicine. The thesis is that if one knows how something happens, one can reason what the effects should be. This approach has been a rich source of hypotheses for testing by clinical research, and many of these hypotheses have been substantiated. This process has provided us with a pharmacopoeia of effective interventions such as vaccines, antibiotics, H2 blockers, and synthetic hormones. But predictions from mechanisms are far from foolproof. In recent years, for example, randomized controlled trials have shown that a drug given to suppress ventricular arrhythmias actually causes death from arrhythmia, and that a vitamin (beta-carotene) given to prevent cancer apparently causes lung cancer. So a sound biologic basis for how an intervention seems to work is a valuable part of the evidence base, but is not decisive evidence for clinical usefulness in its own right.

Interpretation Based on Expert Opinion The best way to incorporate the scientific strength of the evidence into guidelines is to have some members who are experts in this aspect of the work, and to ensure that all members understand enough about the rules of evidence to discuss them intelligently. It certainly is not good practice to defer to panel members with imposing credentials or passionate arguments.

Expert opinion, not explicitly attached to research evidence but rather as an appeal to experience and authority, is often offered as a basis for guidelines. Surely experience provides an invaluable perspective. But for most chronic diseases, even the most extensive personal experience is severely limited for the purpose of drawing valid inferences. There are usually multiple, interacting causes; the effect of any one cause is small and takes a long time to develop, and the same causes can have other effects. Well-conducted clinical research is the right way to understand these relationships.

Expertise in the interpretation of clinical research is a special skill, certainly not highly developed during most medical education and not necessarily associated with special clinical expertise. It is acquired, as other skills are acquired, by reading, discussing, criticizing, writing, and doing research oneself.[9,10] Physicians who are otherwise highly respected in their field might vary greatly in their understanding of the basic principles on which the validity of research conclusions is based. Fortunately, expertise in this area, variously called "clinical epidemiology," "critical appraisal," and "evidence-based medicine," is ever more widely understood and practiced.

HOW IS THE OVERALL STRENGTH OF THE EVIDENCE SUMMED UP?

The strength of the evidence might be characterized by the best existing studies or the totality of the evidence from all reputable sources. The preceding section discussed the strength of research studies taken one at a time. However, important decisions are not ordinarily based on one or another study, but on the totality of the evidence that bears on a question. How, then, is the evidence summed up? Several approaches have been taken.

Results of the Best Clinical Research Studies

Some studies convey a disproportionate amount of the information bearing on a clinical question, sometimes more than all the rest put together (figure 3-3). Much research conducted on animal models and in the laboratory does not produce results that are ready to be applied directly to the care of patients. Of all research on patients, only some is credible,

FIGURE 3-3. The Scientific Value of Different Kinds of Articles

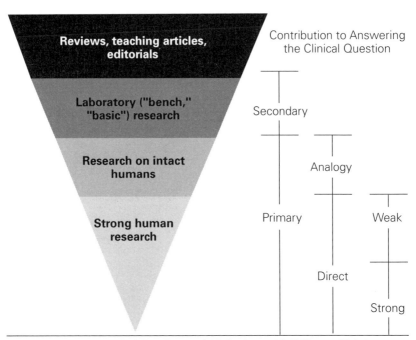

Reprinted, with permission, from R. H. Fletcher, S. W. Fletcher, and E. H. Wagner, *Clinical Epidemiology: The Essentials*, 3d ed. (Baltimore: Williams and Wilkins, 1996).

and a few of the studies are so large and well designed that they should in themselves determine clinical practice. For example, the first randomized controlled trial of screening for colorectal cancer, which involved 45,000 people screened for 13 years, ended decades of uncertainty, when the argument for screening was based on reports of series of screened patients, studies of the sensitivity and specificity of the screening test, and reasoning from the pathogenesis of this cancer.

Systematic Reviews

The results of any one randomized controlled trial, however well done, can be a misleading basis for clinical policies because of the kinds of patients selected for study, biases that have remained undetected, or the play of chance in that particular study. "Systematic reviews" are an increasingly popular way of dealing with the evidence on a single question when a number of scientifically strong studies are available but it remains uncertain what they are telling us. The basic elements of this approach are as follows:

1. Make special efforts to identify all studies bearing on the question, whether or not they are published.
2. Select the studies that meet basic criteria for scientific strength (for the effectiveness of an intervention, well-conducted, randomized controlled trials).
3. Summarize the findings of the individual studies, with the observed effect sizes and confidence intervals.
4. Decide, by statistical methods and good sense, whether the studies are similar enough to one another (in people studied, intervention, and outcome) to be reasonably considered studies of the same question.
5. If they are similar, pool the results of individual studies, as if they are all part of the same study, and the results differ by chance alone, and present a pooled estimate of effect, which is more precise than for any of the component studies.
6. If the studies are apparently not comparable, simply show their individual results or summarize them using a statistical technique that takes into account that their results differ not just by chance, but also because they are addressing different questions.

If it is possible to include data for individual patients, rather than just the summary results of individual studies, then the researchers can examine subgroups of people with special characteristics to see whether the intervention has different effects in different kinds of people. For example, a systematic review of antiplatelet drugs and cardiovascular disease was able to show that men and women respond similarly to the drugs, contrary to earlier thinking in this field.[11]

Bradford-Hill Criteria

The British epidemiologist Sir Austin Bradford-Hill proposed in 1965 that the case for or against a causal hypothesis is the sum of all of the evidence, both epidemiologic and biologic, bearing on the question (table 3-1).[12] Thus, the case is in trouble if we are not sure that the purported cause precedes the effect and if the observed effect is relatively small, since it could be the result of undetected biases. On the other hand, one can draw confidence in finding the same effect in different kinds of people in different places, circumstances, and times. Note that there is no perfectly explicit method for summing up the evidence in this way. It is a value judgment by well-informed, broad-minded scientists.

Rating Systems

Some guidelines groups have established schemes for grading the evidence. This approach is especially useful when a large number of conditions is being considered. The best known is the one used by the U.S. Preventive Services Task Force, an adaptation of one developed by the

TABLE 3-1. The Bradford-Hill Criteria

Criteria	Comments
Temporality	Cause precedes effect
Strength	Large relative risk
Dose-response	Larger exposures to cause associated with higher rates of disease
Reversibility	Reduction in exposure associated with lower rates of disease
Consistency	Repeatedly observed by different persons, in different places, circumstances, and times
Biologic plausibility	Makes sense, according to biologic knowledge of the time
Specificity	One cause leads to one effect
Analogy	Cause-and-effect relationship already established for a similar exposure or disease

Reprinted, with permission, from R. H. Fletcher, S. W. Fletcher, and E. H. Wagner, *Clinical Epidemiology: The Essentials*, 3d ed. (Baltimore: Williams and Wilkins, 1996).

Canadian Task Force on the Periodic Health Examination (table 3-2). The strength of the recommendation for each condition this group considered was graded from A to E, based on "systematic consideration of three criteria: the burden of suffering from the target condition, the characteristics of the intervention, and the effectiveness of the intervention as demonstrated in published clinical research."[13] For the latter, the quality of the evidence was judged by the best available scientific evidence (table 3-3). The quality of the evidence and the strength of the recommendation are not necessarily related; some interventions are known to be effective in cooperative patients but there is good reason to believe that most patients will not accept the intervention.

TABLE 3-2. U.S. Preventive Services Task Force Rating of Strength of Recommendations

Strength of Recommendations

A. There is good evidence to support the recommendation that the condition be specifically considered in a periodic health examination.

B. There is fair evidence to support the recommendation that the condition be specifically considered in a periodic health examination.

C. There is insufficient evidence to recommend for or against the inclusion of the condition in a periodic health examination, but recommendations may be made on other grounds.

D. There is fair evidence to support the recommendation that the condition be excluded from consideration in a periodic health examination.

E. There is good evidence to support the recommendation that the condition be excluded from consideration in a periodic health examination.

Reprinted, with permission, from Report of the U.S. Preventive Services Task Force, "Guide to Clinical Preventive Services," 2d ed. (Baltimore: Williams and Wilkins, 1996).

TABLE 3-3. U.S. Preventive Services Task Force Rating of Quality of Evidence

Quality of Evidence

I: Evidence obtained from at least one properly randomized controlled trial.

II-1: Evidence obtained from well-designed controlled trials without randomization.

II-2: Evidence obtained from well-designed cohort or case-control analytic studies, preferably from more than one center or research group.

II-3: Evidence obtained from multiple time series with or without the intervention. Dramatic results in uncontrolled experiments (such as the results of the introduction of penicillin treatment in the 1940s) could also be regarded as this type of evidence.

III: Opinions of respected authorities, based on clinical experience; descriptive studies and case reports; or reports of expert committees.

Reprinted, with permission, from Report of the U.S. Preventive Services Task Force, "Guide to Clinical Preventive Services," 2d ed. (Baltimore: Williams and Wilkins, 1996).

HOW WILL THE PANEL DEAL WITH SITUATIONS IN WHICH MEMBERS AGREE ON THE EVIDENCE BUT DISAGREE ON THE ACTIONS IT IMPLIES?

Guidelines do, after all, involve value judgments and not just a mechanical application of scientific evidence, leading the panel where it must go. The scientific process is intended to find unbiased answers to factual questions. In their day-to-day work, scientists are used to thinking that the main threat to scientific validity is in the design, measurement, and analysis of data; so might the guidelines panel. But science and its interpretation are a very human enterprise. For example:

- Panel members might be looking at the same numbers but see them differently. The same numbers have different meaning if they are summarized differently. Patients respond differently to the prospect of having a 5 percent chance of dying or a 95 percent chance of living. A 14 times greater risk of lung cancer in cigarette smokers seems like a bigger problem than a risk of 1 per 2,000 people per year, though both summary statistics are based on the same data. Moreover, people in general tend to interpret risks in an illogical fashion—cigarette smokers might fear asbestos in a school, though the risk of lung cancer from smoking is 10,000 times greater.[14] Also, individuals vary greatly in the weight they attach to specific risks. Past experiences and beliefs of those who do science and those who interpret it affect what they see in it—a phenomenon called the "theory dependence of observation." A way to develop a common understanding of the data is to examine data in several different ways (for example, as a relative risk of death, absolute risk, and number needed to treat to save one life).
- Recommendations require more than evidence of effectiveness. They involve value judgments based on evidence, and the "right" course of action rarely simply follows from the evidence itself. Thus, a 1 in 100 chance of finding a treatable disease might be well worth looking for in one person's opinion and a waste of time and money in another's. Evidence-based practices advocated in well-accepted guidelines in one country might not even be considered in another. To deal with this issue, panel members should get in the habit of making a clear distinction between evidence and value judgments and accept that both play a part in recommendations.

FOR WHOM ARE THE GUIDELINES WRITTEN?

They are certainly not written just for the panel members themselves, or for other experts who might admire the elegance or complexity of the work. Average patients, and average clinicians, are implicitly the target of most guideline efforts, though they are too often forgotten along the way.

The guidelines panel must wrestle with a scientific information base that is not well suited to its purposes. Most published research is done by highly specialized academic physicians working in a referral hospital where an unusual selection of patients is seen. The research itself usually excludes, in the interest of getting a clear answer, patients with atypical manifestations of the disease in question, other diseases, or a tendency not to follow medical advice. Researchers tend to choose "hard" outcomes— that is, easily measurable phenomena such as death, persistence or recurrence of disease, or laboratory abnormalities—and to avoid "soft" phenomena such as pain, dyspnea, nausea, or fear. When it comes to complications, researchers tend to report favorable experience and are understandably reluctant to reveal their failures.

On the other hand, most physicians work in less highly selected settings and might be less accomplished than the leaders in their field. Their patients usually have other diseases in addition to the one in question, and express the disease by a full spectrum of possible manifestations. They and their patients care about all the outcomes of care, not just the ones that researchers are best at measuring and, of course, their patients do not always follow their advice!

Panels that wish to base guidelines on scientific evidence, and that are producing advice for the ordinary practice of medicine, are in a bind. The worst resolutions are to pretend that the studies at hand do in fact represent ordinary practice, or to implicitly write the guidelines for the most favorable situation. The best resolution is to carefully locate the studies examined on the continuum from ordinary practice to highly selective referral centers, give special attention to studies from ordinary settings, and make reasoned judgments about how studies from highly selected settings can be generalized.

DO GUIDELINES CHANGE CLINICAL PRACTICE?

Guidelines are intended to improve clinical practice. In modem terms, this means promoting for all members of a defined population the use of clinical practices that have been shown to achieve the best outcomes of care with available resources. How successful are guidelines in achieving this objective?

Guidelines could have their effects on practice at two levels: the process of care and the outcomes of care. The process of care concerns what clinicians do to and for patients, such as educate them and get them to follow advice. Process is a means to an end, not an end in itself. Outcomes of care are the end results, those that patients might especially value such as relief of pain, remission of cancer, or fewer episodes of infection. The main advantage to using process over outcomes of care, which probably accounts for its wider use, is that process can be measured more quickly and easily.

For some care, there is enough evidence linking process to outcome that it is fair to substitute one for the other. Thus, we know that lowering blood pressure (a process measure) prevents stroke and that influenza immunization in the elderly prevents pneumonias and death. We are therefore on sound ground in claiming success when we have increased these processes. But it is not appropriate to substitute process for outcome when a link between them is not known for sure, such as in claiming that it is worthwhile to lower p32 antigen in patients with HIV infection when it is not clear that this leads to fewer infectious complications or longer survival.

There is strong and consistent evidence that clinical guidelines change clinical practice. In a systematic review of 59 published evaluations of clinical guidelines that met criteria for scientific rigor, most of which were randomized trials, all but 4 detected improvements in the process of care and 9 of 11 studies of the outcomes of care reported improvement.[15] However, the magnitude of the effect is another question. In most of the studies, the effects were not large. It seems unlikely that guidelines alone would make large, sustained changes in clinical practice because there are too many other influences on clinical practice, such as patient expectations, practical difficulties, financial incentives and disincentives, and social norms.

Cost was not reported as an outcome of care in these studies, as is typical of the medical literature at that time. Most guidelines have been designed to improve the quality of care without regard to the economic cost. However, the two are not separable in most systems of care and they may be traded off against each other. In one study, proposed guidelines for the use of radiographs for early diagnosis of low back pain would increase utilization over usual care—lumbar radiographs during the first visit would rise from 13 to 44 percent of visits, an increase of 238 percent.[16]

HOW CAN GUIDELINES BE MORE EFFECTIVE IN CHANGING PRACTICE?

Of all the questions discussed in this chapter, this is the most important. Three ways to improve guideline effectiveness in terms of changing clinical practice come to mind:

1. Combine them with other interventions on clinical practice that push practice patterns in the same direction. Among these are

local opinion leaders, education of patients, change in the conditions of a practice to make it easier to do the right thing, feedback on practice patterns, and financial incentives and disincentives.

2. Make them attractive to users. Media specialists have a lot to offer here. Readers are influenced not only by the words in the text but also by brevity, use of color and space, and illustrations.

3. Make them accessible to users. This requires not only a brief, synoptic version but also dissemination in multiple media (the web, print summaries, journal articles, etc.) to suit various users' preferences, gaining attention from the popular leaders, and enlisting the support of local clinical opinion leaders.

Surveys of clinicians in practice suggest that many are not aware of even widely disseminated guidelines and that their attitudes and behaviors are heavily influenced by other factors such as specialty and age.[17] Clinicians have both positive and negative feelings about practice guidelines. In one study, internists recognized the benefits of practice guidelines but were concerned about their effects on their clinical autonomy and satisfaction with clinical practice, as well as the costs of health care.[18] They were much more confident in guidelines prepared by their own specialty society than by an insurer or government. Recent graduates and physicians on salary had more favorable attitudes.[19]

There is much more to be learned about how to make relevant, credible guidelines, how to make their existence known to practicing clinicians, and how to present them in ways that change clinicians' behaviors for the better, in the face of many other influences on practice patterns. I think of guidelines, with the evidence and rationale on which they are based, as a necessary but not sufficient element in the overall effort to improve health care. Now let us move on to the next step, dissemination and learning.

QUESTIONS FOR STUDY

1. Who should be on a guideline panel?
2. What six questions are relevant to evaluating the effect of an intervention recommended by a guideline?
3. What is the advantage of considering unpublished, carefully done research?
4. Name two strong and two weak research designs.
5. What are two major factors affecting study validity?
6. What place does "usual practice" and "mechanism of disease" have in assessing intervention effect?
7. What are the three methods for summarizing evidence?

8. Why might guideline developers make different recommendations based on the same evidence?
9. What are common orientations of well-done scientific studies that lead to their being far from an ideal basis for guidelines?
10. What are some proven and unproven effects of guidelines?

The answers to these questions can be found in Appendix B.

References

1. S. W. Fletcher, "Whither Scientific Deliberation in Health Policy Recommendations?" *N. Engl. J. Med.* 336 (1997). 1180-3.

2. R. H. Brook, "Implementing Medical Guidelines," *Lancet* 346 (1995): 132.

3. M. G. Kortepeter "MRI: My Resonant Image. Letter," *Ann. Intern. Med.* 115 (1991): 749-50.

4. E. A. Codman, "The Product of the Hospital," *Surg., Gyn. and Obstet.* 18 (1914): 491-6.

5. S. W. Winawer, R. H. Fletcher, L. Miller, F. Godlee et al., "Colorectal Cancer Screening: Clinical Guidelines and Rationale," *Gastroent.* 112 (1997): 594-642.

6. S. N. Goodman, J. Berlin, S. W. Fletcher, and R. H. Fletcher, "Manuscript Quality before and after Peer Review and Editing at Annals of Internal Medicine," *Ann. Intern. Med.* 121 (1994): 11-21.

7. P. J. Easterbrook, J. A. Berlin, R. Gopalan, and D. R. Matthews, "Publication Bias in Clinical Research," *Lancet* 337 (1991): 867-72.

8. S. B. Soumerai, T. J. McLaughlin, D. Spiegelman, E. Hertzmark, G. Thibault, and L. Goldman, "Adverse Outcomes of Underuse of Beta-Blockers in Elderly Survivors of Acute Myocardial Infarction," *JAMA* 277 (1997): 115-21.

9. R. H. Fletcher, S. W. Fletcher, and E. H. Wagner, *Clinical Epidemiology: The Essentials,* 3d ed. (Baltimore: Williams and Wilkins, 1996).

10. D. L. Sackett, R. B. Haynes, G. H. Guyatt, and P. Tugwell, *Clinical Epidemiology: A Basic Science for Clinical Medicine,* 2d ed. (Boston: Little, Brown Co., 1991).

11. Antiplatelet Trialists' Collaboration, "Collaborative Overview of Randomized Trials of Antiplatelet Therapy I. Prevention of Death, Myocardial Infarction, and Stroke by Prolonged Antiplatelet Therapy in Various Categories of Patients," *BMJ* 308 (1994): 81-106.

12. A. Bradford-Hill, "The Environment and Disease: Association or Causation?" *Proc. Royal Soc. Med.* 58 (1965): 295-300.

13. Report of the U.S. Preventive Services Task Force, "Guide to Clinical Preventive Services," 2d ed. (Baltimore: Williams and Wilkins, 1996).

14. B. T. Mossman and J. B. L. Gee, "Asbestos Related Diseases," *N. Engl. J. Med.* 320 (1989): 1721-30.

15. J. M. Grimshaw and I. T. Russell, "Effect of Clinical Guidelines on Medical Practice: A Systematic Review of Rigorous Evaluations," *Lancet* 342 (1993): 1317-22.

16. N. E. Suarez-Almazor, E. Belseck, A. S. Russell, and J. V. Mackel, "Use of Lumbar Radiographs for Early Diagnosis of Low Back Pain. Proposed Guidelines Would Increase Utilization," *JAMA* 277 (1997): 1782-6.

17. S. R. Tunis, R. S. A. Hayward, M. C. Wilson, H. R. Rubin et al., "Internists' Attitudes about Clinical Practice Guidelines," *Ann. Intern. Med.* 120 (1994): 956-63.

18. *Ibid.*

19. R. Czaja, S. L. McFall, R. B. Warnecke, L. Ford, and A. D. Kaluzny, "Preferences of Community Physicians for Cancer Screening Guidelines," *Ann. Intern. Med.* 120 (1994): 602–8.

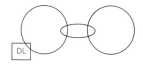

Disseminating and Learning to Use Guidelines

Carmi Z. Margolis, MD, MA

D
issemination and learning comprise the second step in the guideline development cycle depicted in the guidelines bi-cycle (see figure FM-1). Now that the penultimate draft of a guideline has been produced, it must be sent to the people who are going to use it. The effective dissemination of a guideline involves two considerations: the actual mechanics of distribution, and the process of helping clinicians learn how to use the guidelines and make them part of their clinical practice decision making.

This chapter addresses these two considerations and discusses how clinicians can learn to use clinical algorithms. It also features the major educational problems that plague clinical learning and explains how guidelines can address them.

MECHANICS OF EFFECTIVE CLINICAL GUIDELINE DISSEMINATION

Guidelines can be distributed by either conventional or electronic mail, or they can be handed out by someone who worked on developing them. Some suggest that the most efficient way to distribute a guideline is to include it in the electronic medical record. The guideline could be presented in its entirety to be read and learned at the clinician's convenience, or it could guide the recording of the patient's problem. It is possible that both of these ways of integrating guidelines into the electronic medical record will be used in the future, but at present, most practices, even staff model health maintenance organizations, do not use electronic records.

Ensuring That the Clinician Receives the Correct Version

Whatever distribution method is used, a key principle is to make certain that the guideline the clinician receives is the authoritative guideline at the location in which he or she is working. Sending out different versions of a guideline at the same time, or at two close times, is confusing and might seriously disturb learning and subsequent guideline implementation.

I thought guideline distribution was a straightforward matter when I was helping to initiate the clinical guidelines program at the Harvard Community Health Plan in 1987. We were very pleased that the process of using workshops to develop guidelines was working better than had been expected. An orange, loose-leaf binder with tabs was sent to all clinicians along with a note indicating that they were now receiving all of the new practice guidelines that had been constructed by their colleagues, and that these guidelines should be reviewed carefully and filed in the binder. I added that the guidelines program would be happy to receive comments. At about the same time the binder was sent out, the first guidelines were introduced in the Harvard Community Health Plan medical director's newsletter. What could be simpler for clinicians than to read the guidelines, place them in the binder for future reference, and begin to use them to manage clinical problems? We quickly discovered, however, that this was not a simple matter.

From the clinicians' feedback we learned that some of them read the guidelines but most did not. Although some clinicians used the binders systematically, most left them empty on the shelves, without inserting even the first guidelines sent. Newer guidelines found their way into the binder only rarely. The program did not initially set out to systematically collect such evidence of guideline useage. Research has shown, however, that simply distributing guidelines is not an effective way of ensuring that they will be used.

If this seems obvious, consider the following, a true story told by Dr. Gary Freed of a simple sort of guideline and its ineffective distribution. This event took place on a national level, but could certainly be relevant to a variety of individuals disseminating guidelines regarding a variety of specialties.

> I was sitting at a seminar of my fellowship program in 1990 listening to a presentation that showed that obstetricians were still performing too many cesarean sections and ignoring the recommendations from the American College of Obstetricians and Gynecologists. Loyal pediatrician that I am, I was bored by the presentation and was leafing through my copy of the American Academy of Pediatrics newspaper under the table. I noticed an announcement that the Haemophilus influenzae, type b (Hib) vaccine for children was now recommended for use at 15 months of age by the American Academy of Pediatrics. I leaned over to my program director, pointed to this announcement, and whispered that even though obstetricians do not do what their College tells them to,

every pediatrician who saw this recommendation from the AAP would follow it right away. He asked why I was so sure and I said I just "knew it— pediatricians always follow AAP recommendations." He countered that if no one had looked at this issue, I should do a study to prove my hypothesis. As an eager young Fellow, I took him up on the idea and developed a questionnaire to look at the rate of awareness and adoption of the Hib vaccine recommendation among all pediatricians in North Carolina. About a month later, I remember it was a Monday, I had defined my sample, prepared the mailing list and developed my questionnaire. The following Wednesday I was to take my questionnaire to the printer. I was having breakfast with my son and reading our morning paper, when I noticed a small article that stated the Hib vaccine was now approved for use in infants at 2 months instead of 15 months of age. I was shocked. This was the first I had heard of this change. I suddenly wondered how many pediatricians and family physicians were going to learn of this development by reading it in their morning newspapers. It made me broaden the focus of my research question. Would these physicians change the way they gave this vaccine based on something they read in the newspaper? I began to wonder whether the manner in which physicians learn of new recommendations affects their adoption of the recommendations. Luckily, my questionnaire was not at the printer yet!

Two weeks later I received a special letter from the American Academy of Pediatrics informing me of the change in the Hib recommendation. However, our subsequent research was to demonstrate that this letter went only to members of the American Academy of Pediatrics. All other providers of child health care—family physicians, non-member pediatricians—were not sent this information. In fact, the American Academy of Family Physicians did not recommend this vaccine until several months later, leaving members of their professional organization in limbo. Those physicians who were later shown in our research to be the least likely to adopt new recommendations were also the ones who were less well connected to official sources of information.

The next new vaccine recommendation for hepatitis B vaccine was also disseminated in fits and starts. Separate recommendations, each differing slightly, were sent by the Advisory Committee on Immunization Practices (ACIP), the AAP, and the AAFP at different times over a period of 10 months. This created considerable confusion among practitioners regarding who was recommending what and when the recommendation was made. A major effect of our research is that now there is a uniform schedule for these three organizations and they issue immunization recommendations jointly.

Considering Who Should Receive the Guideline

A key principle of dissemination is to consider who should receive the guideline. If, for example, you are going to implement a pharyngitis guideline in a primary care practice or clinic, the clinician is only one of the people who should be aware of and study the guideline. Other providers who should be contacted might include the nurse, the secretary, and anyone else whose job will be affected by the guideline. When teaching nonclinicians how the guideline works, it is usually useful to teach as much of the guideline, including the clinical logic, as the learner can understand. The better the person's sense of the clinical significance of the guideline and how his or her job is facilitating helping the patient, the more chance that he or she will facilitate guideline use.

An often forgotten guideline recipient and participant in any guideline system is the patient. But explaining the guideline to the patient almost never disturbs the care process. It almost always helps. It is true that complex decisions based on knowledge of pathophysiology are usually not the domain of the patient. Even so, some patients might have a scientific background or might take such a strong interest in decisions affecting them that they will learn even highly technical material.

To give one example, I will tell you about an unforgettable patient who I saw when I was a medical student; she had both systemic lupus erythematosis and rheumatoid arthritis. She was intelligent—an artist by profession—and would routinely brief new house officers on all aspects of her disease, including the circulating antibody that had been named after her. She would also refer them to appropriate papers in the medical literature. Clinical decisions, no matter how trivial, were never made without her full understanding, consent, and active participation. This extremely ill woman in her 20s, with her considerably shortened life expectancy and a crippling disability, had a rare disease and great motivation to study it. Most patients will not spend nearly as much time and effort on understanding their disease and its management as did this woman.

Nor will they be as anxious as the surgeon with terminal carcinoma of the colon who was once a patient of mine. He put in his own intravenous lines because he didn't trust the house staff to not hurt him. Patients who have deep understandings of and involvement with fields of science might exhibit abhorrence of disease or be so upset at their condition that they cannot behave rationally.

Contrary to the belief of many clinicians, however, many patients can understand quite a lot about the decisions that will affect their life when the clinicians take the time to explain these concepts. Explaining a clinical decision to the patient not only ensures that we clinicians do not make decisions against the patient's wishes but also maximizes compliance in a way that authoritarian decision making never can.

LEARNING TO USE GUIDELINES

If a guideline is distributed effectively but never learned, its systematic implementation will be severely impaired. From the clinicians' point of view, learning to solve a clinical problem is a central purpose of a guideline. Because we have noted that guideline logic is algorithm driven, learning the clinical algorithm logic that drives the guideline is key to learning any clinical practice guideline.

Learning a conceptual approach to a clinical problem is itself a complex cognitive process that involves at least two kinds of learning: conceptual learning and transferring this learning to solving a practical problem. Educational psychologists call this latter sort of learning "transfer of training." The relationship between learning concepts and transfer of training is similar to the relationship between learning a guideline and using it to guide patient care. It is possible to learn a concept but not transfer it to a practical situation, or resolve the practical problem that involves a certain concept without knowing the concept. It is also possible to learn a guideline but not use it, or to work according to a guideline without understanding it.

Clinical guidelines tend to elicit a negative reaction from clinicians who view them as prescriptions for care and feel they are being told how to practice. However, guidelines are not prescriptive practice recipes at all, but are instead primarily learning maps.

For example, when I was serving as a pediatrician in the U.S. army, my professional hobby was putting together a book of clinical algorithms for the management of newborns. One day at lunch break, Dr. Gray, an experienced pediatrician recently returned from a long tour in Italy, came into my room and read over my shoulder. Dr. Gray had made it clear that he considered himself a consummate practitioner of the medical arts, but that things academic, though interesting, were largely irrelevant to his practice. I was preparing myself for some playful sarcasm when suddenly he said, "Carmi, that's just the way I think about clinical problems. Could I borrow all of those—what do you call them, decision trees?—for the evening?" He read them all one night and returned them with the terse comment, "Great review of neonatal!" Dr. Gray's compliment is one that I have treasured. More than just stroking my ego, it let me know that physicians in practice, like me, thought algorithmically at least part of the time.

Algorithmic Thinking in Clinical Practice

Algorithms are the logic engines that drive clinical practice guidelines. Algorithms describe the usual approaches to mapable problems—that is, problems about which there is general agreement on the approach to diagnostic and therapeutic management. Pharyngitis, diabetic ketoacidosis, and thyroid nodule are examples of this sort of problem. However, algorithms do not deal with certain areas of practice, such as caring for patients or performing the physical examination, and they do not even deal with all of the cognitive part of practice. Other important thinking mechanisms, such as Lawrence L. Weed's problem-oriented problem-solving, pattern recognition, or indeed the pathophysiologic approach to solving a rare problem are not algorithmic, though they may make use of algorithms in the same way that a mathematician solving complex problems may use arithmetic algorithms.[1] Still, at least 80 percent of the problems of admitted patients can be worked up using step-by-step, agreed-upon, algorithmic approaches to management. Residents as well as practitioners of any medical specialty would be lost without them. Teaching clinical guidelines, then, powered by their algorithmic logic engines, can be viewed as teaching a large part of medical practice.

Essential Elements of Algorithm Learning

From the point of view of Jerome Bruner, noted cognitive psychologist and educational theorist, if one can define the nature of the subject, then one can choose an appropriate way to teach it. If an important part of decision making in medical practice is algorithmic, then the educational question is, "How can one best teach clinical algorithms?"

When we first started to investigate algorithm learning in 1972, the answer seemed simple. If one presents the clinical algorithm logic clearly in a flowchart format, then the learner will learn simply by reading it. Today, it is clear that this answer lacks necessary detail. Remember the comparison in chapter 1 of the prose version of the capital gains tax algorithm (exhibit 1-2) and the strikingly clearer flowchart version (figure 1-4)? The point was that it is difficult to use prose to present an algorithm accurately. However, surprise at this realization might obscure a different, more subtle but no less important observation that we all experience, but are not at first aware of, when we read the capital gains flowchart. An algorithm flowchart is sparser in graphics but is dense in information. As we use a particular flowchart branch to solve a problem, step-by-step, we read the branch much more slowly than we would read text or even a list of instructions. We apply the conditional logic to our problem gradually and in small increments. Notice that as we saw in the birthday guessing game (figure 1-2), when you read an algorithm you are not only reading but also using it.

This sort of analysis of how we learn algorithms leads to the following conclusions about how we learn to use clinical practice guidelines:

1. You learn a guideline by using it to solve a clinical problem.
2. Using a guideline involves following each of its logical branches to reach a solution.
3. At each decision point, you must decide whether the patient's data fit.
4. If in your clinical judgment the appropriateness of any guideline decision comes into question, then suspend its use until you decide whether to do the following:

    a. Consult another clinician about the problem.
    b. Use a different guideline.
    c. Merge the inappropriate guideline with another one so that the combined guideline is appropriate.
    d. Stop using the guideline. Use another problem-solving strategy.
    e. Stop using the guideline. You are stumped.

The exercise at the back of this chapter provides a demonstration of how to learn a clinical algorithm using a number of pharyngitis problems.

EDUCATIONAL PROBLEMS THAT PLAGUE CLINICAL LEARNING

We have seen that guidelines describe an important part of the cognitive part of practice and are best learned by first reading them and then using them to solve clinical problems. These characteristics make guidelines especially well suited to addressing the following basic educational problems that have plagued clinical learning:

- Medical practice is still frequently taught as diseases.
- Relevant literature is not linked to clinical practice.
- Essential clinical skills are not well taught.
- Learners do not experience the core set of clinical problems in a discipline.
- Self-instruction and self-evaluation are underemphasized.

The following sections cover each of these problems and explain how guidelines address them.

Medical Practice Is Still Frequently Taught as Diseases

As we write this, a myriad of new, ever more specialized textbooks are being published and sold. Almost all of them, including major textbooks like *Harrison's Principles of Internal Medicine* and *Nelson's Textbook of Pediatrics,* are arranged according to diseases. Most of the vast number of medical journal articles are also about diseases. Years of medical school are spent learning from lectures on diseases and their pathophysiology. Yet we now know that much of this disease-oriented knowledge is not relevant to clinical decision making. Relevant clinical studies, moreover, often are not taught, not properly analyzed, or not linked clearly to the appropriate clinical decision. How to make decisions, solve problems, and improve decision making frequently is not taught at all.

Guidelines address this basic educational problem by presenting information that describes not diseases but practice: decision approaches, with their annotated rationales, are linked to the diagnosis and therapy of specific clinical problems.

Relevant Literature Is Not Linked to Clinical Practice

Should we then stop teaching about diseases and pathophysiology to clinical students and teach only as much science as is necessary to understand guidelines? Not at all. A clear understanding of the basic medical sciences, such as molecular biology, physiology, clinical epidemiology, and behavioral and decision sciences, is still the best basis for understanding health and disease. This sort of understanding maximizes flexibility in clinical problem solving. However, no amount of learning the pathophysiology of asthma will enable the clinician to learn the practical approach to diagnosing and treating acute asthma.

Guidelines address this basic educational problem by presenting carefully analyzed clinical data, such as data on frequency of causes of a problem in a given population or data from therapeutic trials, that are directly relevant to diagnostic and therapeutic decisions. A carefully annotated guideline provides relevant pathophysiology or clinical science at the place the clinician needs it—linked to the relevant clinical decision.

Essential Clinical Skills Are Not Well Taught

Some years ago, a study performed in a quality pediatric residency program showed that when judged by defined criteria, more than 40 percent of the residents did not know how to perform as basic and common a procedure as a tine test. Residents in internal medicine frequently feel that they have little systematic training in as common an area as dermatologic diagnosis; pediatric residents might finish training without learning how to do a proper orthopedic examination of the feet; surgical residents might get minimal training in suturing; psychiatry residents might never learn systematically how to do a psychiatric interview. Medical students might have even larger lacunae in skills learning. There are two reasons for these deficiencies:

1. There has been a failure to define a core of necessary skills appropriate to the clinical level of the learner.
2. Even when a necessary skill is identified, a systematic approach to teaching involving defined criteria and supervised practice frequently is not used.

In contrast, a clinical practice guideline can be read not only as a map of essential clinical decisions, but also as a guide to which skills are necessary to make those decisions. For example, if a urinary tract infection guideline requires the clinician to ask about frequency and dysuria in order to define the problem and to examine unspun urine for bacteria in order to strongly suspect the diagnosis, then by defining these two decisions the guideline also specifies as essential these history-taking and laboratory skills. The teaching of these skills can also be facilitated by electronic enhancement of a guideline, as discussed later in this section.

Learners Do Not Experience the Core Set of Clinical Problems in a Discipline

During the 1960s and early 1970s, medical educators and cognitive psychologists hypothesized general problem-solving strategies that enabled all clinicians to solve clinical problems. However, research in medical problem solving and decision making, both in classroom and real settings, did not suport the central role of general medical problem-solving strategies. By the 1980s, it had become clear that competence in solving clinical problems depended on knowing a large variety of approaches to a range of clinical problems. A competent internist, for example, should know the approaches to the 20 most common problems presenting in adults and, in addition, the approaches to another 20 less common problems. It follows that an internal medicine residency program should provide supervised experience in learning the approaches to solving at least 40 care problems. In other clinical disciplines, the same core of clinical problem approaches should be defined and taught. However, not infrequently, residents complete their training without learning some of these approaches.

Following are examples of situations in which learners, whether students or residents, find they have not experienced the full range of clinical problems that arise within a discipline and of possible ways of dealing with these situations.

Lack of Emergency Clinical Management Training among New Personnel When I began my pediatric internship in the first newborn special care unit in the United States, I was terrified! Although I had done well in my pediatric clerkship rotation on a busy service at Bellevue Hospital in New York City, I felt embarrassingly unprepared to examine newborns with meconium aspiration, idiopathic respiratory distress syndrome, sepsis, and various other common newborn problems that were to me rare or unheard of. Even the most common problem of all, jaundice, somehow had not made it to my pediatric clerkship (perhaps because I never rotated through the nursery?). My panic resulted not only from my never having learned skills such as placing umbilical catheters, but also from having no cognitive approach to managing these clinical problems.

A second incident occurred much later in my career. I became visiting professor at the University of North Carolina at Chapel Hill. While on rounds one day, I was presented with an 11-year old who had chronic diarrhea and over 30 medical problems, and who had been worked up many times at the National Institutes of Health and at North Carolina Memorial Hospital, the main teaching and referral hospital of the university. Most of the patients were similarly complex. When I asked where the house officers had learned to manage common diarrheal illness, pneumonia, and acute bacterial meningitis, I was told that they learned about common problems at an affiliated community hospital. I was immediately reminded of Israeli residents who have the opposite problem. They manage many patients with all the common clinical problems, but hardly ever see epiglottitis, a dangerous disease they must learn to manage, but which is rare in Israel.

These incidents raise two central questions:

1. Is there a way to give early, nonthreatening training in emergency clinical management to new personnel?
2. Is there a way to ensure that clinical trainees will learn to manage a minimum or core set of clinical problems in order to gain basic competence?

Both of these problems can be partly solved by teaching clinical guidelines using simulations that enable the learner to imagine themselves in the clinical situation. In the first scenario above, had I worked through a set of appropriate guidelines and matching simulations, I would have been better prepared to face the newborn special care unit. I would also have had a set of appropriate tools to refer to. Similarly, simulations would have enabled the university residents in the second scenario to at least learn and practice an approach to caring for common pediatric problems, even though they are actually caring for rare problems at North Carolina Memorial and have not yet done a rotation in the community. Simulations would have enabled the Israeli residents at least to partly experience epiglottitis and apply a systematic management approach, even if they were to complete their residency without seeing one real patient suffering from epiglottitis.

Missing Clinical Experiences General surgical residents are required to keep a record of the types and numbers of operations they have done. At the end of their residency, the American Board of Surgery can determine whether or not a candidate has had sufficient experience to allow him or her to perform any of the operations defined to be within the competency of a general surgeon. However, no such system is in effect for medical specialties. No one keeps track of the number of cases of pneumonia, croup, or Henoch-Schoenlein's purpura that a pediatric resident has seen, or the number of cases of asthma, thyroid nodule, adult respiratory distress syndrome, or cancer of the prostate that an internal medicine resident has seen. Although one can usually assume that in the course of a residency on a moderately busy service residents will see enough cases of common illnesses to learn basic diagnostic and therapeutic management, even this assumption might not be correct if the service admits mainly referral cases. Conversely, busy community medical services might rarely see unusual cases. Compounding this problem is the recent tendency to manage in a primary care setting medical problems that formerly were cared for in a hospital.[2] In short, it is certainly possible for a medical resident to complete training without actually having managed a defined variety and number of cases.

Lacunae in management experience might not be picked up by current examinations, because usual examination techniques measure knowledge as opposed to skills or judgment. The candidate therefore can seem to make up for deficiencies in practical experience by studying a textbook or an article.

One solution to the problem of missing clinical experiences seems obvious: The medical specialties must define the clinical curriculum in terms of types and numbers of problems that the clinician learner at any level is expected to see, and must then monitor the learner's experience with managing the problems that comprise the defined curriculum. A complementary solution would be to provide a standard set of simulated experiences that covers the defined curriculum. Standardized patients who teach skills and computer simulations that teach cognitive management approaches are two basic kinds of effective clinical simulations. Bear in mind this important caveat: We do not intend to imply in any way that such simulations would take the place of clinical experience, only that they could complement it either by providing some cognitive experience until the learner managed a patient with the problem, or by serving as a more real review of management than can be provided by a textbook.

Limited Familiarity with Acute Clinical Problems among Inexperienced Residents Another sort of missing piece of clinical experience is relative and temporary, rather than absolute and permanent. Inexperienced residents starting busy intensive care rotations have limited familiarity with acute clinical problems requiring incisive, quick, life-and-death decisions that they will have to make from the day they start the rotation. In recent years, the public has become more aware of the risk of being seen in a hospital in July, when many of the house staff are inexperienced. This problem is dealt with inevitably by throwing more responsibility on the shoulders of the senior house staff, until the juniors gain enough experience to function more independently.

A more satisfactory solution might be to let inexperienced clinicians practice using a set of common, acute, intensive care clinical problems before they begin their intensive care rotations.

Self-Instruction and Self-Evaluation Are Underemphasized

Carl Singer, a family physician and primary care internist who practices in rural New Hampshire, has explained to me that updating clinical knowledge is not a problem for him. His main method is to set aside several hours of work time each week to read journals. What a simple solution! Instead of traveling back and forth to hear an hour of grand rounds esoterica or to attend a course that covers much material he knows well, Dr. Singer uses office time to design and learn from his own reading program. A valid tool for measuring his progress is also available to Dr. Singer in the seven yearly recertification examinations of the American Board of Family Medicine.

Shift from Passive to Active Learning Although clinicians spend most of their learning time teaching themselves, until recently medical schools taught them to learn passively. Lectures and classroom discussions that aim to transfer facts and cover a defined amount of content and laboratory exercises that lead to known conclusions prepare students for summative examinations that emphasize recall.[3] This learning model is so powerfully indoctrinated that despite their discovering that clinical learning takes place primarily at or near the bedside and not in the lecture hall and the classroom, physicians still expect that the truth will be preached from a lectern. No wonder medical students taught in this way expect that as physicians they will learn from review update courses that consist mostly of lectures. Until recently, the continuing medical education establishment has fed this unrealistic expectation by providing a huge volume of officially approved review lecture courses, and only a relatively small amount of experimental self-instructional material.

These officially sanctioned trends toward passive learning and summative evaluation can be reversed only when the establishment clearly signals a shift toward approval of active learning and formative evaluation. As has happened repeatedly when specialty boards have been founded in the United States and abroad, the shift in motivation for, and in quality and content of, learning is sparked by a shift in examination standards. Just as the founding of a specialty board says to the prospective candidate and to the specialist teachers that there is now a body of learning in that specialty defined by a standard examination, institutionalization of relicensure and recertification surely will lead to more appropriate ongoing self-learning and self-examination methods. A sharp shift in the policies of the American Academy of Pediatrics and the American

Board of Pediatrics occurred about 15 years ago with the decision to emphasize learning from an academy-sponsored, continually updated review journal *(Pediatrics in Review)* that routinely provides the reader with self-quizzes. At the same time, the American Board of Pediatrics debuted voluntary and then mandatory periodic, self-administered, computerized recertification. These organizations, among others, have taken leadership roles in spearheading the medical learning revolution.

Role of Electronic Media in Self-Instruction   Electronic media can play a critical role in making self-instruction the basic learning method of the future. We have discussed how a carefully constructed guideline can be used as a learning map that identifies the core set of clinical, problem-oriented decisions of a discipline that are linked to relevant scientific knowledge and clinical skills. When presented in hypertext[4] and hypermedia[5] format on a CD-ROM, a guideline becomes a living teaching system. The electronic format enables the guideline logic map to grow from a flat, two-dimensional guide to a three-dimensional knowledge tree that the learner can climb at his or her own pace, and whose fruits can be picked as needed. Specific advantages to an electronic system include the following:

- The algorithm map that drives guideline logic can be read in any order and to a depth of detail determined by the reader.
- Video and audio enhancement of clinical data allows teaching skills highly relevant to practice. Such skills cannot be taught by text alone. For example, if the guideline presents the differential diagnosis of a murmur, the learner can listen to it. Or if an explanation of seizures directed to a parent is critical to proper seizure management, the learner can, at the click of a mouse, access a video clip that shows an expert explaining to a parent what a seizure is.
- The learner can practice solving clinical problems using a systematically designed set of patient management problems that make him or her use all the logic branches of the guideline.
- An autograding, multiple choice question, self-examination allows the learner to quickly assess whether he or she has grasped the scientific principles and knowledge that provide the rationales for the guideline decisions.
- Other skills-learning modules relevant to the guidelines central clinical problem can be linked to the guideline. For example, a module for learning to read chest roentgenograms has been linked to an electronic version of an asthma guideline. Similarly, a dermatologic diagnosis module could be linked to the electronic version of a guideline for diagnosis and management of rash, or an electrocardiogram diagnosis module could be linked to a chest pain guideline.

PROBLEMS AND EXERCISES

Using a Guideline to Solve Clinical Pharyngitis Problems

Carefully read the template 1988 upper respiratory infection algorithm in figure 4-1 and as many of the annotations in exhibit 4-1 as interest you.

Now, using figure 4-1, try to solve each of the problems in exhibit 4-2. On a separate sheet of paper, write your answers indicating (1) the path you would follow through the guideline (using the box numbers) and (2) the outcome or end point you reach (usually defined by the content of the final do-box in the pathway).

Solutions to these problems and exercises can be found in Appendix B.

References and Notes

1. L. L. Weed, *Medical Records, Medical Education and Patient Case* (Cleveland: Case-Western Reserve University Press, 1969).

2. G. T. Moore, S. D. Block, C. B. Style, and R. Mitchell, "Reply to Somlyo AP. Problem Based Learning: Is It Worth It?" *Acad. Med.* 70 (1995): 341.

3. Summative examinations are end-stage hurdles, like final course exams or licensing examinations, that must be passed before one can reach the successive stage. In contrast, formative examinations provide feedback and might be taken repeatedly until the examinee has learned everything tested by them.

4. Hypertext is a technique for presenting information, now familiar from CD-ROM encyclopedias, in which each flagged term in the text is expanded in a lower layer. The depth to which these layers extend is, in principle, infinite. Another way to view this is as a set of hierarchical linkages between segments of text.

5. Hypermedia, now familiar from electronic encyclopedias and pronouncing dictionaries, establishes similar hierarchical linkages between text segments and audio or video data segments. Astonishingly, hypertext and hypermedia were first proposed conceptually by Vannever Bush in 1945. His idea was to present knowledge in pictures, in sound segments, and in discrete text segments on cards or microfiche. The reader/user would access these materials mechanically in any order at a convenient speed. Today, it is obvious that this was an idea whose technology had not yet been invented.

FIGURE 4-1. Upper Respiratory Infection

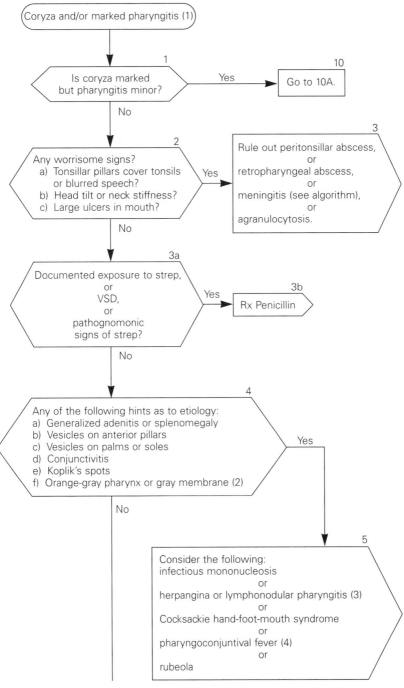

(Continued on next page)

FIGURE 4-1. (Continued)

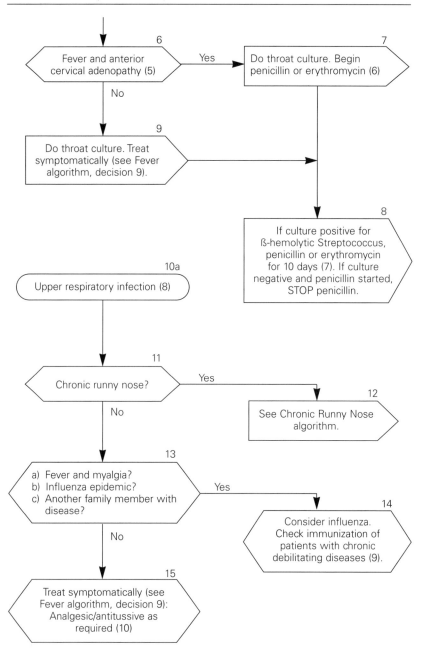

EXHIBIT 4-1. Annotations for Upper Respiratory Infections

1. Although some degree of pharyngitis may be present in coryza, pharyngitis is defined here as a separate entity. The reason for this is the problem of ß-hemolytic streptococcal pharyngitis and its potential complications. We also recommend that throat cultures are done in all cases of moderate pharyngitis, as is explained in Note 5 below.

2. An orange-gray color recalls Tangiers disease(!) (see *Nelson Textbook of Pediatrics*. Edited by Behrman, R.E., and Vaughn, V.C. III. Philadelphia, W.B. Saunders, 1987, p. 343) while a gray membrane suggests diphtheria.

3. Lymphonodular pharyngitis is characterized by nonconfluent vesicles on tonsillar pillars and is thought to be caused by Coxsackie A-10 (see *Nelson Textbook of Pediatrics*. Edited by Behrman, R.E., and Vaughn, V.C. III. Philadelphia, W.B. Saunders, 1987, p. 693).

4. Pharyngoconjuntival fever is an epidemic viral syndrome characterized by intense conjunctivitis and fever (see *Nelson Textbook of Pediatrics*. Edited by Behrman, R.E., and Vaughn, V.C. III. Philadelphia, W.B. Saunders, 1987, p. 682).

5. Despite numerous efforts to diagnose ß-hemolytic streptococcal pharyngitis clinically as described by Breese (*Am J Dis Child* 131:514–517, 1977), there is no convincing evidence that ß-hemolytic streptococcal pharyngitis can be diagnosed clinically unless very strong presumptive evidence of streptococcal infection is present (e.g., another child with proven streptococcal infection in the family or signs of scarlet fever). Moreover, in children less than 1 year of age, streptococcal pharyngitis is uncommon. However, Komaroff and co-workers (*Nurs Res* 25:84–89, 1976) showed that, using the criteria of cervical adenopathy and/or prolonged sore throat, 33% of patients with streptococcal infection were treated early, and only 2% were treated inappropriately. It seems clear that an attempt to prove streptococcal cause using a laboratory test is necessary. Although antigen detection tests have become more common, Gerber and co-workers (*J Pediatr* 108:654–658, 1986) have shown they have a high false-negative rate, thus missing many significant streptococcal infections.

6. If there is a suggestive history of penicillin allergy, such as signs of anaphylaxis or rash clearly related to penicillin, then erythromycin should be prescribed.

7. A positive culture does not reveal whether the patient is a carrier or has an acute infection; therefore, all patients with positive cultures with the clinical picture described here should be treated with antibiotics. Despite the fact that a throat culture should have a false-positive rate of zero. Glass and co-workers (*JAMA* 240:2651–2652, 1978) showed a 60% failure of house staff to identify ß-hemolysis (five times the false-negative rate of the antigen test described in Note 6) and 58% failure to identify a zone of bacitracin inhibition when compared with the judgment of an experienced microbiologist. Thus, if

(Continued on next page)

EXHIBIT 4-1. (Continued)

physicians want to read their own cultures for rapid diagnosis, they must improve their skills and check the validity of their diagnoses.

8. According to Henderson and co-workers (*J Pediatr* 95:183–190, 1979), there are no exact criteria for the diagnosis of bronchitis in children. Our guidelines are URI with cough, usually fever, perhaps with rhonchi, but without signs of pneumonia.

9. We may soon have quick techniques for diagnosing influenza according to Grist (*Br Med J* 1(6009):581, 1976). However, making a strongly presumptive diagnosis using clinical and epidemiologic criteria, viral cultures, and titers will alert clinicans to the fact that, compared to coming down with a cold, the patient may be facing a long course of more severe illness and an increased risk of pneumonia. Also, although it is too late to immunize a patient already diagnosed, the first patient in the autumn with influenza should serve as a reminder to check who in a practice deserves influenza vaccine by virtue of being at increased risk of adverse consequences from infections of the lower respiratory tract (i.e., patients with congenital heart disease, disordered lung function, chronic renal disease, diabetes mellitus, chronic severe anemia, and conditions that compromise the immune system (see Clinical Note in *Clin Pediatr* 19:775–776, 1980)).

10. Use of cough syrup in pediatrics is discussed in detail by the American Academy of Pediatrics Committee on Drugs (*Pediatrics* 62:118–121, 1978). Remember, antitussives do not speed up the course of a viral illness, and they only work when they have a significant cough suppressant effect, in which case they also have more side effects; so, try not to use them. However, if a nonproductive cough seriously disturbs sleep or school performance, prescribe codeine or dextromethorphan. But remember that doses for use of the drugs are not based on firm data in children; the available data suggest a low therapeutic ratio for codeine; symptomatic treatment may mask underlying disease.

EXHIBIT 4-2. Case Examples—Upper Respiratory
Infection Algorithm

For each of the following cases, record the algorithm pathway used and
the outcome according to the algorithm.

Case 1
A 22-year-old man presents with two days of runny nose and slight cough,
and has today begun to have fever to 101 degrees Fahrenheit with
occasional chills and muscle aches. He has taken aspirin once. Physical
examination is unremarkable except for temperature 100, mild pharyngitis,
and clear rhinitis.

Answer: Pathway:
              Outcome:

Case 2
A 12-year-old girl comes to you with two hours of sore throat and fever.
On physical examination, her temperature is 102, and her left tonsil is
not visible. You notice that she answers questions as if her mouth is full
of food.

Answer: Pathway:
              Outcome:

Case 3
Arlene, a 30-year-old woman, tells you her throat hurts since this morning
and she feels feverish. Her 6-year-old son had streptococcal pharyngitis
demonstrated by culture three days ago. On physical examination she has
moderate pharyngitis and slight tenderness of a right anterior cervical node.

Answer: Pathway:
              Outcome:

Case 4
Tony, a 42-year-old bisexual man who has been perfectly well, presents with
a stuffed nose, a sore throat, and a severe cough. On physical examination,
his temperature is 100, his respiratory rate is 28, and he is slightly labored;
his lungs have fine rales over the entire left side. The other exam is
unremarkable.

Answer: Pathway:
              Outcome:

Case 5
George, an 18-year-old, comes in complaining of feeling sick, having a mild
sore throat, and a 100-degree temperature for a day. On physical
examination, he has severe pharyngitis with a few petechiae on his uvula,
exudate on his erythematous tonsils, but no cervical adenitis.

Answer: Pathway:
              Outcome:

(Continued on next page)

EXHIBIT 4-2. (Continued)

Case 5a

What if George had the same presenting symptoms, but on physical examination also had a tender left anterior cervical node?

Answer: Pathway:
             Outcome:

Case 5b

George's culture shows no growth. What now? Consider both case 5a and case 5b.

Answer: Pathway:
             Outcome:

Case 6

Art, a large 5-year-old, presents with a sore throat and decreased appetite over three to four days (his mother isn't certain). On physical examination, there are moderate pharyngitis with some exudate; very prominent bilateral anterior cervical nodes; and palpable occipital, inguinal, and axillary nodes. A spleen tip is palpable.

Answer: Pathway:
             Outcome:

Case 6a

What if Arthur had no nodes on physical examination but had vesicles on his palms and soles?

Answer: Pathway:
             Outcome:

Reprinted, with permission, from *Designing Care Coursebook*, published by the Institute for Healthcare Improvement, Boston, © 1991–1996.

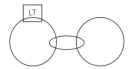

5

Tailoring Guidelines

Carmi Z. Margolis, MD, MA

The third and last step of the development cycle in the guidelines bi-cycle is local tailoring. Chapter 6 begins discussion of the second wheel of the guidelines bi-cycle—the implementation cycle.

This chapter defines local tailoring and uses a fictitious case to illustrate the usefulness of the guideline tailoring process. It also discusses the three factors that might necessitate local tailoring and gives a global example of local tailoring.

LOCAL TAILORING

Local tailoring, or customization, of a clinical practice guideline is the process of enabling clinicians and other patient care personnel to make changes to an authoritative guideline to make it more suitable for practice in a particular clinical setting. Two central aims of local tailoring are as follows:

1. To enable local personnel to gain guideline ownership
2. To facilitate implementation

Tailoring changes might affect diagnostic or therapeutic decisions. They are not changes in evidence-based guideline decisions. Rather, they are changes that will suit the guideline to differences in local disease prevalence, system of care, or other local peculiarities, such as use of a particular drug or laboratory test. Efficient methods for tailoring are the same nominal group process and Delphi process techniques used for achieving consensus during the process of guideline development (see chapter 2). Local tailoring might be viewed as a final iteration of the consensus process used to develop the guideline.

The Case of Dr. Maatsch

Dr. Art Maatsch is a family practitioner who also heads the clinical guidelines program in a large, southern health maintenance organization called SuperCare. A few weeks ago, when his six-year-old son, Jamie, was treated for his first bad asthma attack, Dr. Maatsch was surprised that his family practitioner recommended adrenaline as a first-line drug. The next day, a pediatrician whom Dr. Maatsch trusts used albuterol. After a two-day hospitalization that included a short course of steroids and cephalexin, Jamie recovered from his attack and returned to school.

Motivated by Jamie's hospitalization, Dr. Maatsch reviewed asthma care at SuperCare and found disturbing data:

- Different primary care physicians are indeed using different treatment approaches. Family physicians sometimes use adrenaline as a first-line drug, but pediatricians usually use inhaled albuterol.
- The measurement of peak flow, which Dr. Maatsch now knows is strongly recommended to determine treatment effectiveness, is rarely done. He himself is not sure how to do it. No attempt is being made to use prognostic categories to predict which patients will need hospitalization, and Dr. Maatsch suspects that too many patients are being put in the hospital.
- Recent data from the pharmacy indicate that large amounts of cephalexin were being used to treat patients with asthma. Examination of the records of a sample of these patients revealed no indication of treatment other than the diagnosis of asthma and the hospitalization itself. Dr. Maatsch remembers that Jamie never had a fever, though he was treated at first with intravenous antibiotics and then with cephalexin.
- Either a clinic visit or an admission for asthma is a common indication for a chest x-ray. Children under six years of age with asthma have had an average of three chest films per year.

Very concerned about these errors in asthma management, Dr. Maatsch convened a guideline committee consisting of the planwide chief of pediatrics, the planwide chief of family medicine, and the chief of nursing services. Dr. Maatsch decided to use the National Heart Lung and Blood Institute's guideline for asthma care, although the chief of pediatrics said something to the effect that the American Academy of Pediatrics' version is more appropriate for children. The chief of nursing services also mentioned that she hoped this new emphasis on guidelines, and especially the peak flow business, didn't end up increasing the work of the already overloaded nurse practitioners (they take lots of time; she used to do them in respiratory clinics). Most worrisome is the response Dr. Maatsch received when he described his plans to a close friend and colleague who works with him in the same practice group. This usually reasonable fellow sympathized with Dr. Maatsch's concerns over the variation in asthma care for children, but added that he was in no mood for more guidelines from above, especially if they would make more work to satisfy some administrator, present company included.

Questions Raised by the Case

Dr. Maatsch's predicament raises several questions that have been dealt with in previous chapters. These questions and their possible answers are as follows:

- Is an asthma guideline needed at all?

Perhaps each of the problems Dr. Maatsch discovered can be dealt with in a specific way without developing and implementing a guideline. To address the problems that he found, Dr. Maatsch might plan a separate approach to each. For example, he could send out a circular suggesting that, and explaining why adrenaline is no longer considered a first-line drug for acute asthma. At the same time he could take adrenaline off the health maintenance organization's pharmacopoeia, except for use in resuscitations. He could then send out another memo requiring all primary care physicians to measure peak flow before and after giving bronchodilators, while at the same time providing peak flow meters in clinics and in the emergency room, and so on. This would be like the proverbial blind men developing a plan for discovering what was attached to the leg, trunk, or ear of the elephant they had got hold of. But it would have been far more effective for the blind men to have asked a seeing person what the elephant was. In the same way it would seem much more efficient and reasonable to adopt a health maintenance organization–wide guideline that would address use of bronchodilators and antibiotics, measurement of peak flow, indications for a chest x-ray, and indications for hospitalization—provided, of course, that the guideline is not only adopted but also implemented.

- How many people and which people should be on the guideline committee?

As discussed in chapter 2, all those involved directly with the care of asthma should be represented on the committee, but the number should be between 7 and 10 people. This might include primary care and specialist physicians, nurses, and administrators directly responsible for asthma care on the ward, in the emergency room, and in the clinic. Should it also include the people responsible for transporting the patients from the emergency room to the x-ray department? It should only if there is a problem with transporting patients.

- Which guideline should be the template for SuperCare's guideline?

The guideline that should be the template is the one most recently developed by a recognized authority on the care of asthma in children. In this case, the seed might be the American Academy of Pediatrics asthma guideline.

- Does the search for evidence have to be repeated?

That depends on how recent the authoritative guideline is. The rule of thumb is that the literature search should be repeated from the end of the search that was the basis for the authoritative guideline. In this case, if the American Academy of Pediatrics guideline was published in January 1995 and the literature search was updated in September 1995, then the local search would begin from October 1995. However, the central question for Dr. Maatsch is, "How should I be dealing with the obvious resistance of administrators and other colleagues?"

LOCAL TAILORING AS A TECHNIQUE TO REDUCE RESISTANCE TO GUIDELINES

Local tailoring is a powerful technique for reducing resistance to guidelines because it enables practitioners to rewrite, or at least critique, the guideline to reflect local input and conditions.[1, 2] For example, a clinician cannot implement a pharyngitis guideline that requires a rapid strep test if his or her emergency room does not have the test available. Tailoring allows you either to change the guideline or, especially if the decision in question is essential, to anticipate modifying your practice environment to enable the guideline to be used properly.

Local tailoring also allows personnel involved with the guideline at different levels in the care hierarchy to feel a sense of guideline ownership. Tailoring enables you to co-opt guideline users in a meaningful way.

At this point, one or more of the following questions might have occurred to you:

- Once the national guideline is tailored for conditions at Super-Care, can this version of the asthma-in-children guideline be used in any SuperCare facility?
- To what extent does an authoritative guideline have to be tailored?

- Is it enough to tailor a national guideline for use at a particular hospital or health maintenance organization, or do you then have to tailor the health maintenance organization version for use by a group within the health maintenance organization, or even for use by a particular practitioner?

The answer to all of these questions is this: It might seem more efficient to implement the health maintenance organization version unchanged at all facilities, but experience shows that if tailoring is more specific, more local, it is more likely that clinicians will use the guideline on a patient-by-patient basis.

Some evidence-based guideline developers might pounce on this point. They would insist, on the one hand, that the reason we base the guideline on evidence is that decisions grounded on hard evidence do not have to be tailored. Restated in proper scientific terms, if the quality of evidence is rated "I" and the strength of the recommendation is rated "A," the decision should always adhere to the recommendation.[3] On the other hand, if a decision is not grounded on evidence, say the evidence is rated "III" ("opinions of respected authorities") and the recommendation is rated "C" ("there is insufficient evidence to recommend for or against. . . but recommendations may be made on other grounds"), then it would be better not to make a recommendation at all, and to let the practitioner suit the particular decision to the patient. Tailor the decision, they would say, rather than the guideline.

In considering this approach, we would first point out that whether or not evidence is the basis for a recommended guideline decision is a guideline development rather than a guideline tailoring or implementation problem. Tailoring is a technique that addresses the problem of how to implement or use a guideline that has already been developed. We agree that if there is good evidence for a decision, it should not be tailored in the guideline. Only in this way can you encourage clinicians to see guidelines as useful tools that they control, rather than as prescriptions they must follow.

LOCAL TAILORING VIS-À-VIS USING THE GUIDELINE TO SOLVE A PATIENT'S PROBLEM— TAILORING THE DECISION TO THE PATIENT

Using a guideline to solve a patient's problem is sometimes referred to as tailoring guideline decisions for the patient. However, this is not the same as local tailoring of guidelines. Using the guideline for patient problem solving has already been discussed in some detail in chapter 4. That discussion is from the perspective of how a physician transfers guideline learning to decision making about real patients. However, since tailoring the decision to the patient is so essential to using guidelines properly, we will revisit this issue from the perspective of a busy clinician who has to make frequent, real clinical decisions.

Factors That Might Cause Deviation from a Guideline Recommendation

Decisions about a patient can deviate from a guideline recommendation because of the following factors:

- Physician factors: Even if we assume that the clinician intends to follow the guideline, a fight with his or her spouse just before coming to the office or lack of sleep, to name only two physician factors, might cause a judgment error.
- Environmental factors: Environmental factors, like urinary red blood cells in a patient with acute glomerulonephritis, are too numerous to count. Examples are the centrifuge breaking in the laboratory so that urinalysis cannot be performed as specified in the urinary tract infection guideline, or the winter flu epidemic causing such an increased patient load on a particular morning that the pediatrician has no time to perform essential parts of the physical examination specified by the well-child guideline.
- Patient factors: These might be unrelated to the guideline, whether or not the guideline is based on evidence. For example, the evidence would dictate treating a nonallergic febrile patient strongly suspected of having streptococcal pharyngitis with amoxicillin, either while awaiting culture results or in the absence of cultures. But if the patient vomits following the first dose and is otherwise drinking well, the clinician might agree either to defer treatment until culture results are received, or to perform cultures that were not done at first.

From this perspective of varying patient factors, it is essential that any guideline decision be viewed only as a guide that is applied after a competent clinician decides that the guideline decision suits the patient. After all, even the best evidence-based guidelines do not manage patients. They can only be used as tools, similar to expert systems, to assist in patient management.

Three Factors That Might Require Local Tailoring

Now that we have discussed solving a real patient's problem—that is, tailoring the guideline decision for the patient—let us consider tailoring the guideline to a local setting. Before the guideline is ready to be given to a clinician, whether or not it is evidence based, some research and much common practice suggest that it might be unsuitable for a particular clinical setting because of three factors:

1. Disease prevalence factors: An example of a prevalence factor is that if pneumococci in a particular region are frequently insensitive to penicillin, another drug recommendation would have to be substituted in the pneumonia guideline.

2. Care system factors: A care system factor for a pharyngitis guideline would be that if a particular rural setting did not have bacterial culture facilities readily available, then all patients with a relatively high clinical probability of strep (for example, fever + unilateral cervical node tenderness) would have to be treated.

3. Local factors: An example of a local factor might be adding to the pharyngitis guideline the trade name of the cheapest amoxicillin locally available in order to encourage its use.

These factors might affect either diagnostic or therapeutic decisions suggested by the guideline. All of these changes can only be tailored by clinicians who will be using the guideline in their own setting. The changes would obviously enhance guideline usefulness and increase local clinician commitment to guideline use.

Nominal group process (discussed in chapter 2) can be used as a tailoring tool to elicit local changes in much the same way it is used to encode expertise and reach consensus when developing the guideline. However, tailored changes almost always reflect local factors rather than change in intrinsic guideline logic.

It is, of course, possible, though unlikely, that a clinician participating in a local tailoring group might have cogent reasons from new literature for modifying a guideline decision. If this evidence supersedes that used by the guideline, then even a basic guideline decision might be tailored. This sort of change should also be communicated to the guideline developers for use in the next guideline draft.

GLOBAL EXAMPLE OF LOCAL TAILORING

The most ambitious example of local tailoring that we know of is the attempt to tailor the World Health Organization's Global Program on AIDS Guidelines for Management of HIV/AIDS in Adults and Children.[4] The adult guidelines were first drafted in May 1989 in an attempt to provide template guidelines mainly for developing countries, but also for developed ones. Developers first thought that when the guidelines were completed they would be taught to public health personnel from different countries who would then help local clinicians modify them for actual use. However, as the developers began to appreciate the importance of local factors, this plan was changed to using nominal group process in order to assist local clinicians in producing a local draft of the global guidelines. After four such drafts were produced, in countries as different as Malawi, Barbados, Thailand, and Burundi, a workshop was held in Ethiopia for representatives of another 18 countries in order to train them in group processing the guidelines for local use. Rigorous comparison of the drafts produced by three of the countries showed that changes fell into the following three categories:

1. Changes necessitated by differing disease prevalence: Disease prevalence had a major effect on tailoring the template global guidelines, since these guidelines made numerous recommendations regarding diagnosis and treatment of malaria in patients with AIDS, but in Barbados and in parts of Thailand there is no malaria.
2. Changes necessitated by differences in the care system: In Malawi, where there were no university hospitals, the care system required that all sections of the template guidelines aimed for use at "Level C" (tertiary care hospitals) be deleted. Similarly, Barbadian clinicians took out all "Level A" sections aimed at clinicians working in the bush with only their stethoscopes, since in Barbados all primary care facilities have much more sophisticated facilities available.
3. Changes necessitated by local factors: Local factors, such as drugs in use in a particular country, accounted for many other changes. Generally speaking, only generic names of drugs were used in the guidelines, but in some cases, where the same drug has two or more generic names (paracetamol/acetaminophen, ampicillin/polycillin, etc.), the local variant was, of course, used in the local draft.

Though clinicians who participated in the workshops expressed almost uniform satisfaction with the consensus process, and local drafts were produced within four months, we unfortunately have no data regarding how these drafts were used subsequently.

You can now see that an authoritative guideline may be developed not only at a national but even at an international level, depending on whether the clinical problem is only a national problem or is also a global one, such as AIDS, homicide, or malaria. However, regardless of the level at which the guideline is developed, it must subsequently undergo one or more tailoring processes that are similar to the consensus process of guideline development. Only then will the guideline be suited for use in a particular clinical setting.

Large countries should pay particular heed to the AIDS global guidelines story, since they generally have variations in disease prevalence and care systems that make them function like a patchwork of smaller countries with varying diseases and care settings. Proper tailoring and implementation of national guidelines might not change these factors, but could limit variation in care quality across differing disease prevalence and care settings.

We believe that local tailoring is practiced by almost all serious guideline users at some point before final implementation. However, it is rarely discussed, and even then not systematically. Little research has been done on the nature of local tailoring changes, which are sometimes referred to with embarrassment, as if this process taints the purity of evidence-based work and should be avoided. We would encourage guideline workers to research the nature of the tailoring process and the changes it produces.

QUESTIONS FOR STUDY

1. What is local tailoring?
2. What are the two purposes of tailoring?
3. What three sorts of differences in the local setting might require changes in an authoritative seed guideline?
4. What sort of methodology is used to tailor guidelines locally?
5. Can local tailoring change a decision firmly based on type I evidence and an "A" level recommendation?
6. How is local tailoring different from tailoring a decision to a patient?
7. Can tailoring be done on any level guideline, or is it limited to guidelines generated at a national level?
8. Is tailoring part of the guideline development process or of the implementation process?

The answers to these questions can be found in Appendix B.

PROBLEMS AND EXERCISES

1. Describe how you would go about tailoring the hyperglycemia guideline of the National Diabetes Association to be used at a large health maintenance organization.
2. How would you plan to use the Agency for Health Care Policy and Research guideline for AIDS management in your AIDS clinic?

Solutions to these problems and exercises can be found in Appendix B.

References

1. L. K. Gottlieb, N. H. Sokol, K. Oates Murrey, and S. C. Schoenbaum, "Algorithm-Based Clinical Quality Improvement: Clinical Guidelines and Continuous Quality Improvement," *HMO Practice* 6, no. 1 (1992): 5-12.

2. S. C. Schoenbaum and L. K. Gottlieb, "Algorithm Based Clinical Quality Improvement," *British Med. J.* 301 (1990): 1374-6.

3. C. DiGuiseppi, D. Atkins, and S. H. Woolf, Eds., "Task Force Ratings," in *Guide to Clinical Preventive Services: Report of the U.S. Preventive Services Task Force* (Alexandria: International Medical Publishing, 1996), pp. 861-85.

4. R. Wabitsch, C. Z. Margolis, J. E. Malkin, K. Abu-Saad, and J. Waksman, "Evaluating the Process of Tailoring the Global HIV/AIDS Practice Guidelines for Use in Developing Countries," *Int. J. Quality HealthCare*, 10, no. 2 (1998): 147-54.

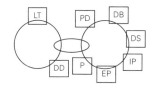

6

Putting Clinical Guidelines into Practice

Shan Cretin, PhD, MPH

This chapter begins discussion of the guideline implementation cycle depicted in the guidelines bi-cycle (see figure FM-1). At the core of this cycle is quality improvement, which in this context refers to the impact of guideline implementation on the quality of care provided by health care organizations. When health care organizations talk about guideline implementation, they sometimes speak of the two different types of implementation interchangeably. The distinction is this: One is implementation of an individual guideline in a practice setting, the topic of this chapter; and the other is implementation of a guideline program, discussed in chapter 8.

This chapter presents strategies for overcoming clinician and administrative resistance to guideline implementation. It also discusses the relationship between guideline implementation and the quality improvement process. Appendix A at the back of this book contains a detailed implementation case study that exercises the principles covered in this chapter.

CONCEPTUAL FRAMEWORK FOR IMPLEMENTING CLINICAL PRACTICE GUIDELINES

Implementing a guideline is similar to implementing any other new program or system in an organization. The organization and the people in it will have to change, and many will resist. Success is difficult, if not impossible, without planning who will do what by when; without budgeting resources to carry out the plan; and without active support for the change by managers, clinical staff, support staff, and patients.

Actually having the elements of the guideline understood and used by the clinical team to guide care begins with the selection of the clinical problem the guideline will address. Implementation of the guideline inevitably requires change to a greater or lesser degree. For those clinicians whose practices differ from those recommended by the guideline, the change required is obvious. However, even those whose practices by and large conform with the proposed guideline might resist the creation of explicit statements about clinical practice unless they see a compelling reason for doing so. The key to successful implementation is to understand and effectively address that resistance from the very beginning of the guideline development process. It is important to remember throughout the process that just because your clinicians automatically hate every guideline, it does not mean that their objections to this particular guideline are groundless.

The change model shown in figure 6-1 provides a useful framework for understanding the elements needed for successful guideline implementation. These elements are as follows:

1. Create tension for change.
2. Identify an effective alternative.
3. Provide social supports.
4. Develop self-efficacy skills.
5. Build a supporting infrastructure.
6. Include a mechanism for feedback and evaluation.

These elements and strategies for dealing with them are discussed in the following sections.

FIGURE 6-1. The Change Model

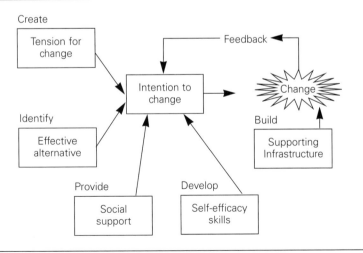

Reprinted, with permission, from *Systems to Support Health Policy Analysis: Theory, Models, and Uses* by David H. Gustafson, William L. Cats-Baril, and Farrokh Alemi (Chicago: Health Administration Press, 1992), p. 45.

Create Tension for Change

Guidelines are hard to implement if the clinicians do not perceive that there is a problem with the current care. Creating tension for change refers to the attempt to help clinicians recognize the need for change. The clinical problem selection process is a way to establish this. Without tension for change, reactions such as the following are likely to greet any proposal for a new clinical practice guideline:

- "I have more serious things to worry about than whether a healthy 45-year-old woman 'feels prepared' for menopause!"
- "We don't need a guideline on pneumonia vaccination. All of my eligible patients are already vaccinated."
- "Why do we need to use warfarin for deep view thrombosis prophylaxis with hip replacement patients? The American Academy of Orthopedic Surgery has no recommendation on prophylaxis method and many of my patients do just fine with unadjusted coumadin."

People feel blindsided if someone else has been documenting and evaluating their performance and then announces changes without having consulted and collaborated from the outset. A collaborative team of providers, support staff, and managers ought to be involved in guideline topic selection and in the collection and evaluation of data on which to base that selection.

When clinicians participate in the process of reviewing their own clinical and cost data and in making comparisons with benchmark facilities, they are likely to agree that change is necessary. The best strategy for inspiring support for change is to collect and report data that reinforce the need for change before introducing the guideline. However, even after a guideline is introduced, asking clinicians to review their own cases relative to the guideline can be a powerful way to illustrate the need for more standardization of practice.

Clinicians often fail to appreciate the degree to which there is variation in practice, and even chart reviews of a relatively small number of cases can help make the point that variation is not just a cost issue. The following two stories illustrate these points: A primary care group practice asked each physician to review the vaccination status of 10 elderly patients seen in the previous month. No physician reported a pneumonia vaccination rate of over 50 percent, which caused a shift in the discussion about the pneumovax guideline from "This is a waste of time" to "How can we improve compliance?" In another example, a large hospital was having trouble establishing the need to reduce the postsurgical wound infection rate because surgeons viewed the 3.4 percent infection as acceptable and within the range of normal practice. Attitudes changed following the circulation of an article from the *New England*

Journal of Medicine that suggested that rates of less than 1 percent are quite feasible,[1] coupled with a report based on a chart review of recent cases: "Out of 25 cases reviewed, we found 12 different prophylactic antibiotic dosing regimens were prescribed. The preop and postop nursing staffs find it difficult to be consistent and punctual in delivering medications to patients with so much variation. At the same time, our postoperative wound infection rate is six times as high as the best reports in the literature."

Keys to Success

- Pick a clinical topic that is important to providers.
- Pick a clinical topic where there is a perceived performance gap.

Operational Tips

- Establish a multidisciplinary team to select the guideline area, defining the patient group and the aims of care for that group in terms of process and outcomes.
- Encourage a collaborative atmosphere that helps to reduce mutual blaming and professional jealousies.
- Encourage a systems view of care delivery to establish a context for the guideline and to highlight the need for coordinated teamwork.
- Provide the team with data on its own performance and access to the literature and other comparative data.
- Better yet, involve the team in the collection and review of its own data.
- Involve patients in focus groups and videotape these to help clinicians see the problems from the patient perspective.

Identify an Effective Alternative

Even when there is agreement that the current methods of caring for patients need changing, clinicians might still resist adopting a new or "seed" guideline because they do not believe it will improve the situation. To be seen as an effective alternative, a guideline needs to be both valid and feasible. To this end, the steps recommended in the guideline design and development process have the following two simultaneous and interrelated goals:

1. To develop the best possible guideline based on the evidence
2. To develop a consensus that the evidence-based guideline recommendations are valid and reasonable in the practice setting; this ensures that clinicians understand and agree on the evidence and also that they agree about the availability of the essential elements needed to follow the recommendations

A new guideline containing many controversial recommendations or ignoring the most recent clinical literature is likely to fail, and deservedly so. However, a technically well-researched guideline might not be seen as an effective alternative if those who are being asked to implement it were not involved in, or at least well informed about, the development process. The process used to select or develop a seed guideline needs to be based on rigorous review of the evidence and open to broad participation by many different providers. Early in the development, it is important to include pharmacists, rehabilitation therapists, nurses, social workers, and others who will be involved in implementing the guideline.

When recently developed guidelines already exist for a clinical topic, the first step should be a rigorous review of these existing guidelines. Established criteria for guideline review, such as those developed by the Institute of Medicine (see table 6-1), are a good place to begin. A detailed method for critiquing existing guidelines is presented in chapter 2.

TABLE 6-1. Characteristics of a Good Clinical Guideline

- Validity
  Correctly interpreting available evidence, so that when followed, valid guidelines lead to improvements in health.

- Reproducibility
  Given the same evidence another guideline group produces similar recommendations.

- Reliability
  Given the same clinical circumstances another health professional applies them similarly.

- Clinical applicability
  Target population is defined in accordance with scientific evidence.

- Clinical flexibility
  Guidelines identify exceptions and indicate how patient preferences are to be incorporated in decision making.

- Cost effectiveness
  Guidelines lead to improvements in health at acceptable costs.

- Clarity
  Guidelines use precise definitions, unambiguous language, and user-friendly formats.

- Multidisciplinary process
  All key disciplines and interests (including patients) contribute to guideline development.

- Scheduled review
  Guidelines state when and how they are to be reviewed.

- Documentation
  Guidelines record participants, assumptions, and methods; and link recommendations to available evidence.

Adapted, with permission, from *Clinical Practice Guidelines: Directions for a New Program*. Copyright 1990 by the National Academy of Sciences. Courtesy of the National Academy Press, Washington, DC.

Review of existing guidelines can help a team arrive at a "seed guideline" more quickly. However, the seed guideline development process is far from over. The "seed" needs to be circulated, and this process of circulating a guideline can also be an educational process for providers. Using a clinical algorithm, or flow diagram, to give a picture of logic behind the guideline is helpful. This clinical algorithm of the guideline can be supplemented with additional detailed annotations, references, and even copies of key articles, including any recent review articles. Key guideline recommendations must be annotated, including references to studies that support the recommendation and an overall grade for the strength of the evidence based on an accepted standard, such as that shown in table 6-2.

Key to Success

- Clinicians agree that the recommendations in the guideline are consistent with the best medical evidence.

Operational Tips

- Develop and circulate a fully annotated and documented "seed guideline" complete with references to the relevant literature.
- Review existing guidelines as a means to "jump start" the development of a good "seed guideline."
- Use a standard method to "grade" the level of support for key recommendations.
- Consider attaching copies of two or three key articles when the "seed guideline" is first circulated.

Tailoring a Guideline to Local Conditions

In some organizations, guideline review can be a perfunctory business. However, merely sending a copy of the guideline to physicians and other providers is no guarantee that the guideline will even be read, let alone

TABLE 6-2. Quality of Evidence

A: Randomized controlled trial with large sample
B: Randomized controlled trial with small sample
C: Prospective trial or large case series
D: Retrospective study
E: Expert opinion
S: Literature summary or formal review
M: Metanalysis
Q: Cost-benefit or decision analysis
L: Legal requirement
X: No evidence

carefully reviewed. Thus, any evidence-based seed guidelines should be submitted to a formal process of local tailoring (discussed in chapter 5) to ensure that the recommendations contained in the guidelines are appropriate to the patient population and feasible in the practice setting.

Evidence-based guidelines are not to be considered as "one size fits all." Rather, they are dependent on the level of training of the provider, the technical capability of the site, and the characteristics of the patient population that interact with care decisions. What is appropriate for asthma care in a middle-class, suburban physician's office is not necessarily appropriate in an inner-city emergency department or a remote health station in the Alaska bush. Guidelines for handling chest pain patients in a university medical center emergency department might call for cardiologic assessments that are simply unavailable at a rural hospital that is part of the same health system.

Because the kinds of issues that arise in tailoring a guideline can be clinical or administrative or both, it is important to ensure that the review process includes a variety of people and uses a range of formal methods. We will return to a detailed discussion of tools for reviewing and tailoring guidelines to local conditions later in this chapter.

Provide, Develop, and Build Support

Although creating tension for change in the selection of the guideline topic and offering an effective alternative in the design of an evidence-based, practical guideline are necessary steps for successful implementation, they are not sufficient in themselves to ensure success. All the components shown in figure 6-1 must be in place: Social support must be provided, self-efficacy skills must be developed, and a supporting infrastructure must be built.

Addressing these last three steps in the change model might be difficult if any of the following critical barriers are present:

- Organizational culture does not support practicing according to the guideline.
- Providers lack the skills and knowledge necessary to practice according to the guideline.
- Patient demands conflict with guideline recommendations.
- Providers forget to follow the guideline.
- Support systems cannot meet guideline requirements.
- Economic incentives are not aligned with guideline recommendations.

These specific barriers and strategies for addressing them are discussed in the following sections.

Organizational Culture Does Not Support Practicing According to the Guideline The lack of support for guidelines in an organization can be general (that is, the very idea of any clinical guideline raises hackles) or specific (for example, the guideline recommends having the anesthesiologist prescribe and administer prophylactic antibiotics when in this organization that has always been the purview of the surgeon). General resistance to guidelines is likely to be more difficult to overcome.

One practical strategy is to identify those providers who are open to guidelines and begin with them. Building on the positive experiences of a receptive group within the organization has a much better chance of success than fighting an entrenched and committed opponent. If only a few orthopedic surgeons are interested in a primary hip replacement guideline, let these pioneers begin the process of implementation and use the feedback and evaluation data to highlight the differences between guideline and nonguideline patients in terms of length of stay, complications, costs, and other key measures.

Another effective strategy is to identify the opinion leaders among the providers and invest in a serious effort to win them over. Arrange for these influential physicians to visit other health care organizations for which guidelines have been used successfully, and let their peers at these sites provide information and answer concerns. Where the lack of support is specific to the guideline, targeted education or changes in particular policies are needed. Existing avenues of communication, such as grand rounds or a medical staff newsletter, can reach a broad audience but might not be as effective as enrolling enthusiasts and opinion leaders to talk with their peers.

Providers Lack the Skills and Knowledge Some guidelines founder because the providers lack the skills to implement them and are unable or unwilling to admit this deficiency. For example, at one medical center surgeons were reluctant to prescribe certain drugs for deep vein thrombosis prophylaxis in their hip replacement patients because these mostly elderly patients had other comorbid conditions or maintenance medications with which the surgeons were not very experienced. Providing easy access to pharmacologic consultations helped to improve the surgeons' skills and provided needed support.

It is useful to review any new guideline to identify the skills and knowledge the guideline will require. Will nurses need to assess activities of daily living? Will physicians need to read chest x-rays in order to distinguish asthma from other pulmonary conditions? If so, prepare training materials in advance and make them available in nonthreatening ways. Computer-aided self-study modules are one way to allow providers to walk through a new algorithm, assess their own performance on sample cases, and select areas for additional training in a safe, private environment. Large multisite organizations like Kaiser–Permanente can marshal the resources to put together a continuing medical education module based on a new guideline, complete with readings, self-study modules, patient education materials, and other supportive materials.

In addition, a guideline resource packet can be supplemented with a technique called "academic detailing." Academic detailing is modeled on "drug detailing," but instead of calling on physicians to introduce a new drug on a one-on-one basis, the "academic detailer" provides information and education about an evidence-based practice guideline. Nurses or other professionals can be trained and supported to answer questions, provide articles from the literature, and explain any new systems that will be used to implement the guideline, such as changes in standing orders or new forms to be incorporated in the medical record. In some organizations, the "academic detailers" revisit the physicians after the guideline is implemented and provide feedback regarding individual and group compliance with key guideline recommendations and patient outcomes. Academic detailing involves the following elements:

- Conduct focus groups to understand current behavior, identify barriers
- Define clear behavioral and educational objectives
- Establish credibility, reference authoritative and unbiased sources, present both sides
- Use concise, graphic educational material
- Highlight and repeat essential messages
- Provide one-on-one education
- Reinforce with feedback

The evidence regarding the effectiveness of clinical education in changing behavior suggests that personalized interventions are more successful than generic mailed materials or grand rounds. Physicians are also more likely to pay attention to educational material if they have received feedback on their personal performance that indicates a gap between their practice and the ideal care.

Patient Demands Conflict with Guideline Recommendations

Clinician education is often most successful when linked with patient education. Physicians need access to materials in lay language that will answer patient questions and correct mistaken ideas that lead patients to insist on tests or treatments that have little or no demonstrated value. In large organizations such as the Veterans Health Administration, it is possible to run focus groups with patients prior to implementing a guideline to learn what their questions and concerns are likely to be. Providing physicians with the answers to "Frequently Asked Questions" on a one- or two-page "cheat sheet" can reduce the stress physicians feel when guidelines ask them to eliminate treatments or tests that are popular with patients.

Providers Forget to Follow the Guideline A key method for encouraging compliance with guideline recommendations is the use of a variety of decision support strategies, the goal of which is to make it easy for providers to do the right thing. At the simplest level, decision supports consist of feedback and reminders. Feedback is most effective when it is individualized, allows private comparisons with group performance (as opposed to public exposure), and comes in a timely manner.

Usually feedback is coupled with a reminder of the desired practice. Not surprisingly, concurrent reminders (those given just as one is about to make a choice) are more effective at changing behavior than retrospective reminders ("Yesterday you did the wrong thing."). In organizations with automated clinical records, reminders can be programmed into the system. Computerized order entry systems can be programmed to suggest the orders recommended by the guideline. Even in paper systems, redesign of encounter and order forms can offer concurrent reminders.

Decision support can also be built into the design of work and the designation of who does the work. For example, changing standing orders and creating detailed pathways can enable nurses in surgical intensive care to safely extubate patients without having to wait for a specific order from a surgeon for each patient. Similarly, training office staff to offer patient education about menopause can ensure that women receive the information they need without requiring the physician to be involved directly in each case.

System Cannot Meet Guideline Requirements A critical factor in the success of any guideline is the assurance that the system can actually support the care required by the guideline. For example, if according to the guideline women need to be biopsied within 24 hours of detection of breast lumps, then the system must be capable of scheduling a biopsy for the day after any day, seven days a week. It is far better to delay the implementation of a guideline until the system is upgraded or improved than to hold physicians accountable for standards they cannot meet due to factors outside their control. Assigning high-priority process improvement teams to key support functions—such as radiology or laboratory testing required by a clinical guideline—is one effective way to address system capability.

Here is an example of a system that could not support its guideline requirements, with tragic results. At a large eastern health maintenance organization, women died after their breast cancers were left undetected. The health maintenance organization lost considerable prestige in the community and several million dollars in justified legal actions. Facing the crisis head on, a medical management team collected data from practitioners and patients that showed that two factors were involved in the mistakes: lack of examining skill on the part of practitioners and patients, and failure to get suspect breast lumps to a surgical clinic quickly enough.

A multidisciplinary team consisting of primary care practitioners, surgeons, nurses, radiologists, and pathologists constructed a well-researched, carefully drawn, and reasoned practice guideline for workup of a breast mass. The central decisions included identifying a suspicious mass correctly and getting such a mass to the breast clinic within one week. An elegant clinical teaching method involving models and supervised breast palpation was used to teach basic skills. A multimedia version of the guideline was made readily available in all adult primary care clinics. The chief of general surgery signed off enthusiastically. However, at first pilot, the guideline failed. Why? There had been no administrator on the guideline team and no administrative review of the guideline. No detailed implementation plan had been written. When the guideline went into effect the general surgical clinic was overwhelmed by breast mass referrals within one week and had to close for a month. A single estimate of referral increase and projection of increased clinic appointment volume could have prevented this.

Economic Incentives Are Not Aligned with Guideline Recommendations Often, the most difficult aspect of implementing a new guideline is addressing the discrepancy between the economic incentives a provider faces and the recommendations in a guideline. For example, in rural China, 80 to 90 percent of a village doctor's income comes from a markup on the sale of drugs. For many conditions, good medical practice requires that the village doctor refer the patient to a higher level where laboratory tests and more skilled providers are available. Changing the payment system to reward good practice (referral, in this case), rather than the provision of inappropriate services (in this case, giving patients intravenous amino acids or prescribing five antibiotics at a single visit), is an essential part of any serious effort to implement guidelines. The clinical situation might not seem as stark in the United States, but perverse economic incentives are pervasive.

Key to Success

- Clinicians and support personnel agree that the recommendations in the guideline can be implemented with the resources and supports available to them.

Operational Tips

- Engage clinical, support, and administrative personnel in the identification of barriers or problems that might interfere with practicing in accordance with the guideline.
- Use tools such as the nominal group process (discussed in chapter 2), force field analysis, and failure mode and effects analysis (discussed in the next section) to encourage in-depth review.

TOOLS FOR GUIDELINE REVIEW AND PROBLEM PREVENTION

An essential step in developing a guideline that is truly capable of being implemented is the identification of possible barriers or administrative issues. A team might find it helpful to systematically review the guideline using more or less formal review tools. At the simplest level, a multidisciplinary team can consider the following two questions:

1. Why are we currently practicing the way we do?
2. Why are we *not* going to follow the guideline?

This process is also called administrative review. One example of a decision not to follow the guideline is this: For a team considering the management of transient ischemic attacks, the obvious reason that so many patients with transient ischemic attacks were hospitalized (current practice) was related to patient preferences. Patients were frightened and wanted the reassurance of being in the hospital. The guideline recommended sending low-risk patients home and prescribing aspirin. Again, patient preferences loomed large as a reason not to follow the guideline. "Here is a patient who is worried that he is having a stroke and you want me to tell him, 'Take two aspirin and call me in the morning!'" If the guideline is to be followed, then before implementation, patient education materials would have to be developed and a system would have to be established for giving patients reassurance without hospitalizing them.

Another way to capture administrative issues is to use managerial tools such as force field analysis and failure mode and effects analysis. While these two techniques will lead to the identification of some of the same factors, they are different enough and easy enough to use so that many teams find it valuable to use both.

Force Field Analysis

Force field analysis encourages a review of the guideline as a whole and helps to identify policies, social norms, legal constraints, educational factors, and economic incentives that might work to facilitate or impede adoption of the guideline. It has been used for many years in planning and managing change. The idea is simple, but powerful: Ask those who will be involved in implementing a change what forces will work with them in promoting the change (driving forces) and what factors will work against them (restraining forces) (see figure 6-2). It is useful to identify a few common categories ahead of time that seem relevant to the problem at hand. In the case of implementing guidelines, relevant categories include patient influences, sociolegal considerations, education and skills, economic incentives, and administrative factors.

FIGURE 6-2. Driving Forces and Restraining Forces

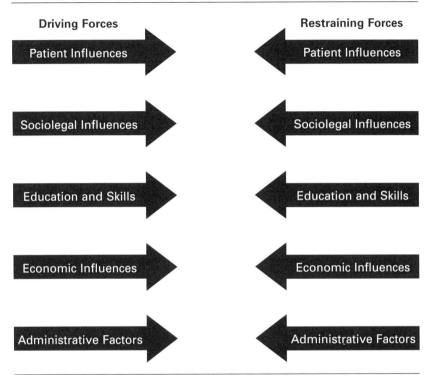

Force field analysis can be done individually, but working as a group is likely to generate more ideas and a shared sense of what needs to be done. Some groups find it easiest to separate brainstorming ideas (with no discussion or comments) from classifying ideas into categories. The classification tends to lead to discussion, which can then shut down the generation of new ideas.

Once a force field analysis has been completed, the team can think about how best to capitalize on driving forces and how to deflect or eliminate restraining forces. Experience shows that success depends on effectively addressing restraining forces, rather than focusing on drivers. If there are too many items for the team to handle, then the team should prioritize the key restraints and address the most critical items. For example, one particular pain management guideline required nurses to assess hysterectomy patients' pain levels within one hour of arriving on the unit and at regular time intervals thereafter. Restraining forces included the following:

- Nurses' belief that these patients did not have significant problems with pain
- Too many demands on the limited nursing time available

Nurses' beliefs about pain were addressed in two ways:

- Sharing results of patient satisfaction surveys showing postoperative pain and inadequate pain medication as major dissatisfiers for hysterectomy patients
- Having nursing students conduct and report on a special postoperative pain assessment for 30 hysterectomy patients, demonstrating that pain was inadequately managed in more than one-third of the cases

Lack of time was addressed by engaging the patients in self-assessment of their pain. First, they were supplied with a clipboard, a cheap electronic timer, and a form on which to chart their pain. Then, patients were instructed about the pain self-assessment as part of the preoperative workup. Finally, they were again reminded about the self-assessment and given the self-assessment kit when they were transferred from the recovery room to the unit.

When force field analysis is used in conjunction with other tools such as failure mode and effects analysis, be sure to collapse the list of problem areas identified by different methods. Affinity grouping is a useful technique for creating a short list of independent problem areas for planning purposes.

Steps in Affinity Grouping

1. Write brainstormed ideas on individual cards or pieces of adhesive note paper.
2. Randomly place cards on a table or place notes on flip-chart paper taped to the wall.
3. Without talking, each person looks for two cards or notes that seem to be related and places these together, off to one side. Others can add additional cards or notes to a group as it forms or reform existing groups. Set aside any cards or notes that become contentious.
4. Continue until all items have been grouped (or set aside). There should be fewer than 10 groupings.
5. Now discuss the groupings as a team. Generate short sentences that describe each group and use these as title cards or notes. Avoid one- or two-word titles.
6. Items can be moved from one group to another if a consensus emerges during the discussion.
7. Consider additional brainstorming to capture new ideas using the group titles to stimulate thinking.

A plan should then be developed for each key barrier or problem area, including the following:

- Who
- Will Do What
- By When
- With What Resources

Failure Mode and Effects Analysis

Failure mode and effects analysis is a systematic method for identifying potential problems in a newly designed product so that the design can be strengthened to prevent, or at least ameliorate, the effects of the most serious problems likely to be encountered. It takes the guideline apart, step-by-step, to identify barriers or problems that might contribute to a lack of compliance. In the classical application of failure mode and effects analysis, the team responsible for the design of, for example, a satellite, looks component by component at the design and, as shown in exhibit 6-1, asks the following:

1. What failure modes could occur?
2. How seriously would each of these failure modes affect the overall performance of the system?
3. What are the possible causes of each of these failure modes?
4. How likely is each of these causes to occur?

Then, from the long lists of failure modes and likely causes, the team can prioritize the most severe failure modes and most likely causes and strengthen the design to avoid or overcome these potential problems.

EXHIBIT 6-1. Failure Mode Effects Analysis Table

Process Step	Potential Failure Mode	Severity (S) (1–5)	Possible Causes	Likelihood (L) (1–5)	Priority (L x S) (1–25)	Overall Effect

From MIL-STD-2070 (AS). *Procedures for Performing a Failure Modes Effects and Criticality Analysis for Aeronautical Equipment,* Washington, DC, Department of Defense, 1963.

A clinical guideline, as a design for delivering medical care, can be subject to the same kind of "preventive engineering." Working alone or in teams, clinicians, support personnel, and administrators can review a proposed guideline box by box to identify failure modes and causes, and to rate the severity and likelihood of the items they identify using the failure mode and effects analysis form that follows.

Let's apply failure mode and effects analysis to an illustrative example: a single box in a more complex guideline pertaining to hip replacement patients—namely, the box relating to antimicrobial prophylaxis.

Administer intravenous cefazolin beginning no more than 2 hours prior to incision and continuing 12 to 24 hours postop.

Step 1. Identify the Failure Modes What are the different ways in which we could fail to comply with this guideline? We are not looking for legitimate exceptions or contraindications, but genuine failures. In fact, following a guideline when one should not is itself a possible failure mode. The failure modes are as follows:

1. No antibiotic prophylactic is administered at all
2. A different intravenous antibiotic is prescribed
3. The correct drug is given, but by a route other than intravenous
4. The correct drug is given by intravenous, but is not started until after surgery
5. The correct drug is given by intravenous, but is started more than 2 hours prior to incision
6. The correct drug is given by intravenous, beginning less than 2 hours prior to incision, but continuing more than 24 hours after surgery
7. The correct drug is given by intravenous, beginning less than 2 hours prior to incision, but is discontinued less than 12 hours after surgery
8. Guideline is followed inappropriately, patient had contraindication

Step 2. Determine How Serious This Failure Mode Would Be Usually, we ask the team to rate each failure mode on a 1 to 5 scale with 1 being "not serious," 2 being "somewhat serious," 3 being "moderately serious," 4 being "very serious," and 5 being "extremely serious." It is easier for people to assign these numbers after they have considered all the different failure modes that might occur. Some teams write each failure mode on a separate piece of adhesive note paper and let the team roughly rank order them on a flip-chart sheet marked with a five-point scale.

In our example, the team may decide that omitting the antibiotic (failure mode 1) or administering a contraindicated drug is very serious, ranking at 4. On the other hand, continuing the drug beyond 24 hours may be seen as not very serious, ranking at 1. Using a different antibiotic might be more difficult for the team to score, since it might depend on which drug is substituted, so the team may assign a range, 2 to 3.

Step 3. Determine the Possible Causes for Each Failure Mode

For example, the antibiotic might not be administered (failure mode 1) because everyone who might have administered the drug thought someone else had already done it (cause A). The same failure mode could also be due to ignorance of the guideline's existence on the part of the clinicians involved with the case (cause B). It is possible that some of the same causes might apply to more than one failure mode. For example, ignorance of the guideline (cause B) could also lead to the wrong drug, wrong route, or wrong timing (failure modes 2 through 8).

Step 4. Determine the Likelihood of Each Cause Occurring

Usually, it is sufficient to rate each separate cause on a 1 to 5 scale with 1 being "not at all likely," 2 being "somewhat likely," 3 being "moderately likely," 4 being "very likely," and 5 being "extremely likely." Some teams choose to anchor the extreme points by first agreeing on which of the causes is most likely and which is least likely and assigning those causes a 5 and a 1, respectively. Other teams simply create a rough rank ordering of causes from most likely to least likely (ties are acceptable), using the technique described in step 2 above. Each cause is written on a separate piece of adhesive note paper and the team places each note at the appropriate place on a flip-chart sheet marked with a five-point scale.

Step 5. Prioritize Failure Modes and Causes for Prevention and/or Amelioration Efforts

A quick-and-dirty way to identify key failure modes and causes is to simply multiply the likelihood by the severity to create a priority score (see the second to last column in the failure mode and effects analysis table in exhibit 6-1), and then pay attention first to those failure modes and causes that contribute to the highest priority scores. For causes that appear again and again in different parts of the guideline and are associated with different failure modes, some efforts at prevention might be warranted, even if the priority scores associated with the problems generated by this cause are generally low. For priority areas, the team can try to prevent (or reduce the likelihood of) the cause, or change the system so that even if the cause occurs, the failure does not.

When faced with an evidence-based recommendation that is not feasible in the proposed practice setting, the team can choose either to change the system of care available so that the recommendation is feasible, or to change the recommendation. Trying to hold providers to guidelines that cannot be implemented is a formula for failure. "I would love to deliver thrombolytic therapy to myocardial infarction patients in the emergency department within 30 minutes of their arrival, but many times I don't even see the patient until 45 minutes after their arrival."

On the other hand, for a guideline to be practical and feasible it is not necessary to address every possible eventuality, no matter how unlikely or obscure it might be. (Remember, a characteristic of the practical guideline is that it does not cover every situation.) Rather, the team needs to identify the critical barriers or problems and address them either by revising the guideline or by establishing a realistic plan for changing the system of care. In the next section, we will consider practical practice support strategies that can be used to overcome the barriers to implementing a guideline.

GUIDELINE IMPLEMENTATION AND QUALITY OF CARE

As mentioned earlier, quality improvement is at the core of the guidelines implementation cycle in the guidelines bi-cycle. The following two sections present a scenario illustrating the need for a guideline to improve the quality of care for asthma patients, and then a discussion of the relationship between the steps in quality improvement and those involved in guideline implementation.

Implementation of a Guideline for Managing Asthma

Not long ago, one of us was asked to consult on implementing an asthma guideline for children and adults in a small health maintenance organization called Healthcorp, which consisted of 25 groups that admitted all their patients to a well-run, 300-bed community hospital that served a city of 350,000 people. Dr. Armand Rhenish, chief of internal medicine, and Dr. Francine Smith, chief of pediatrics, were convinced that emergency room and clinic practice were far too variable across physicians in the various groups. Some pediatricians were using inhaled beta-2 agonists every 10 minutes for children in acute distress, while others administered them every 20 minutes. There seemed to be no agreement as to how many times they should be used before making a decision to admit. Dr. Smith also felt that the sequence of drugs used in the practices was quite inconsistent. I asked whether she thought the variation in drug use had economic implications. She said she thought that one of the drugs was much more expensive than a generic that the health maintenance organization preferred, but they had not been successful in getting the pediatricians to use the generic.

She also said that three months ago one older pediatrician had used subcutaneous epinephrine as a first-line drug for an eight-year-old boy who presented to her practice in acute distress, with a respiratory rate of 60 and almost absent breath sounds. Although the epinephrine was given in the correct dose, the child's pulse went up to 190 and he vomited several times immediately after the shot. Within seven minutes his breathing was much more relaxed and his respiratory rate was down to 35. However, the parents, one of whom was a bioengineer working at the hospital, insisted that epinephrine was the wrong drug and that their child had been subjected to unnecessary side effects. They were now suing the hospital.

Dr. Rhenish explained why he felt the internists needed a guideline for managing asthma: "You see, there is no question that they should be using peak flow measurements to monitor how the patients are doing. For some time now, peak expiratory flow is recommended in the literature as a key measure of pulmonary function in obstructive lung disease, and it is clear that rapid improvement of peak flow predicts how well the patient will do after discharge from the emergency room. But our physicians are not using peak flow measurements—neither in the clinic nor the emergency room! Just yesterday, one of them had the chutzpah to tell me that he could judge patients' clinical status quite well without forcing them to undergo a "very uncomfortable procedure" that gets them even more out of breath!

These two energetic and positive physicians then told me that they had already planned out a "program of more than 10 guidelines that have to be implemented over the next year." I asked what their administrative support was like, both at the level of the chief administrative officer of the health maintenance organization and of the hospital and at the level of the groups.

Dr. Rhenish, somewhat surprised at my question, said, "Oh, well we can certainly get them to do what we want. After all, they are facing a major suit about that child. I'm sure they will agree to improving clinical care!" Dr. Smith added, "The nurse in our practice is terrific. She'll do anything I ask her to."

Asked whether she thought that there ought to be special consideration given to teaching the guideline and disseminating it, Dr. Smith said she supposed so, but figured that the difficult part was getting the guideline developed and distributed. If the guidelines were good, she was certain that most pediatricians (and internists for that matter) would use it. Dr. Rhenish agreed, but wanted to have some more formal evaluation of whether the guideline was being used. He thought that the medical records personnel could take care of that. They both felt that they needed help with guideline implementation and wanted to get started as soon as possible.

Quality Improvement Process

Using a guideline to improve quality of clinical care is similar to improving any other work process. Quality improvement, for example, improving wait times or the quality of telephone answering procedures, should proceed in the manner shown in table 6-3.

In the table, the steps of the usual quality improvement process have been indicated in parallel to those of the guideline implementation process. Notice that the steps of the two cycles of the guidelines bi-cycle (see introduction) all appear. If we now assess Healthcorp's guideline implementation intentions, we might come up with the following analysis:

1. Project definition: Dr. Rhenish and Dr. Smith present a convincing case that Healthcorp has significant asthma care problems that can be corrected by implementing an asthma guideline. These include a possibly incorrect process of asthma care resulting in legal entanglement, as well as the cost of certain bronchodilators. However, there are not enough data to be certain what the nature and extent of these problems are. Data should be collected on the use of peak flow meters in the emergency room, types of beta-2 agonists used according to physician, and other malpractice suits related to asthma care.

TABLE 6-3. Quality of Care Cycle

Process improvement	*Clinical improvement*
1. Project definition	1. Project definition
2. Diagnostic journey	2. (Hi-level process flow diagram)
	Develop guideline
	Detect failure modes
3. Remedial journey	3. Develop decision supports
	Write implementation plan
	Disseminate guideline
4. Evaluation and feedback	4. Implementation and evaluation
5. RETURN TO STEP 1.	5. RETURN TO STEP 1.

2. Diagnostic journey: It is unclear whether Dr. Rhenish has already chosen an asthma guideline, but it is definite that he has one in mind. The same is true for Dr. Smith's asthma-in-children guideline, although she mentioned the American Academy of Pediatrics guidelines several times. Therefore, there is no need to develop an asthma guideline, because excellent ones have been developed recently. However, Dr. Smith and Dr. Rhenish must choose specific guidelines and then must initiate a local tailoring process.

3. Remedial journey: Presently there is no strategy for learning, disseminating, or implementing the proposed asthma guidelines. Drs. Smith and Rhenish seem to have only a vague notion of what dissemination or implementation involves. They are relating to both administration and nursing personnel as subordinates in a hierarchy rather than as members of a team. Therefore, dissemination and implementation processes will have to be planned and effected.

4. Evaluation and feedback: Again, Dr. Rhenish has not thought much about the difficulties involved. He does not see evaluation as his problem, but rather as a technical issue that he would like solved by others. Therefore, an evaluation plan will have to be developed and effected in parallel to the implementation plan.

Is the level of sophistication of these guideline implementation problems characteristic of implementation problems in most care facilities? We have not gathered data that would allow us to answer with certainty. However, we can say that from our experience these problems are not unusual.

SIGNIFICANCE OF THE IMPLEMENTATION PLAN

In many health care organizations, the prevailing culture reinforces the notion of the physician or surgeon as the single individual responsible for what happens to patients. In reality, the quality of medical care delivered to patients is rarely, if ever, the result of the action or decisions of one single individual. Good care and good patient outcomes depend, instead, upon the coordinated efforts of skilled teammates.

For example, in many hospitals, each surgeon is allowed to dictate the preferred operating room setup and postoperative care regimen for each procedure he or she performs. This degree of customization is justified by the belief that the surgeon is the most important determinant of the success of the surgery, and that any efforts to force surgeons to standardize their work would degrade their performance. However, the consequences of this customization policy are far reaching: the setup process for the operating room is complex, hence increasing the chance of errors and delays in setup; the inventory of surgical supplies includes many minor variants of similar items requiring more storage space, more complex retrieval systems, and increased chance of running out of a particular item; and training of operating room techs, scrub nurses, and recovery room staff members is complicated by the need to learn many different protocols and surgeon preferences.

Having a single deep vein thrombosis prophylaxis protocol following hip replacement or a single guideline for postsurgical extubation of cardiac patients might force a particular surgeon to change his or her practice, but the development of consensus around these items will make it easier for the rest of the clinical care team to coordinate their care. It is also easier to identify and prioritize the system resources that need to be mobilized. Therefore, it is possible to draw the following axiom and corollaries.

- Axiom: A guideline is a valuable framework for organizing and coordinating the care given by a team of providers.
- Corollary: Guidelines can help identify system resources that need to be mobilized, and prioritize the needs for improvement in support processes such as pharmacy, lab, and admitting.
- Corollary: Guidelines can help identify and prioritize needs for continuing medical education and skill development.
- Corollary: Guidelines can be the basis for improved communication about patient care among different caregivers.

For these reasons, clinical guidelines are too important a tool for improving patient care to allow them to be adopted in name only. Every guideline needs an implementation plan to ensure its implementation and ongoing evaluation as part of a continuing program of clinical improvement.

Reference

1. Classen, et al., "The Timing of Prophylactic Administration of Antibiotics and the Risk of Surgical Wound Infection," *New. Engl. J. Med.* 326, no. 5 (1992): 281-6.

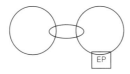

7

Evaluating and Monitoring Clinical Practice Guidelines

Shan Cretin, PhD, MPH

E valuation and monitoring are integral to the meaningful use of guidelines as tools for clinical improvement. The problem is selecting what
to evaluate and what to monitor, keeping in mind that the purpose is
not biomedical research but effective, consistent, day-to-day clinical practice. These monitoring and evaluation decisions seem to come at the end
of the guideline development and implementation process. However, to
be successful, the choice of measures and the design of the evaluation
need to be integrated into the beginning of the guideline process, and
into the actual selection and tailoring of the guidelines.

This chapter provides a framework for the evaluation and monitoring process. It also offers 10 steps to consider when attempting to effectively measure guideline evaluation and monitoring.

FRAMEWORK FOR THE EVALUATION
AND MONITORING PROCESS

A useful framework for selecting measures to evaluate and monitor the
effects of a guideline on patient care considers the impact of inputs (such
as patient characteristics) and processes of care on the outcomes of interest (clinical outcomes, patient satisfaction, and, inevitably, cost and
resource use) (see figure 7-1). This framework suggests the domains that
need to be considered in selecting measures, but we need to find other
principles that help us identify a few essential variables necessary for two
types of guideline assessment:

- Initial evaluation of a newly introduced guideline
- Ongoing evaluation of the effects of a guideline via a practical, parsimonious monitoring system

These principles are discussed in the following sections.

Initial Evaluation

When a guideline is first introduced, evaluation has the following multiple purposes:

- To understand (and address) the barriers to implementing the guideline
- To see whether the care recommended by the guideline is actually followed and actually improves outcomes
- To decide whether to modify the guideline, abandon the guideline, or continue to use the guideline on a routine basis

A rich, dynamic set of measures is needed to conduct this type of formative evaluation. The "bottom line" in guideline evaluation is to assess the impact on patient outcomes. However, in the early stages of guideline implementation, it makes sense to first ascertain the degree to which guideline recommendations are, indeed, being followed. To this end, input and process measures might be needed to evaluate adjustments to the guideline, the implementation approach, and the support systems. Because formative evaluation is a dynamic process, specific measures might be introduced to shed light on a particular problem area and then dropped when the problem is resolved. For example, in implementing a guideline to improve pain management following surgery, if patients' pain is not being assessed in a timely manner, resulting in delays in titrating pain medication, one can temporarily monitor the number of cases for which no pain assessment was done within two hours of admission to the unit. Once pain assessment is routinely carried out, the measure can be dropped.

FIGURE 7-1. Framework for Selecting Measures

Input	Process of Care	Outcomes
Patient characteristics	Test ordering	Mortality and morbidity
Qualifications of providers	Treatments	Functional status
Location of service	Timing of events	Patient satisfaction

Ongoing Evaluation

Once the value of the guideline and the support systems have been established, ongoing monitoring of a very small number of measures will help to maintain effective control and alert us to changes or possible problems.

The primary purpose of this monitoring phase is to see whether the outcomes continue at the same level. The best measures to meet this purpose are usually end-result outcomes, such as the percent of patients reporting adequate pain control. Sometimes the end-result outcome measures are difficult to obtain, in which case the most effective monitoring strategy might be to focus on proximate outcomes (blood pressure control, rather than numbers of strokes over the next five years), or even process measures (percentage of vaccinations against pneumonia, rather than pneumonia cases). A secondary purpose of ongoing monitoring might be to ensure that a few (very few!) key elements of the guideline continue to be followed.

Figure 7-2 shows the relationship between the evaluation and monitoring activities and the effects on measurement. If the ongoing monitors show a sudden drop in the effectiveness of pain management, or if a new drug needs to be incorporated in the pain management guideline, we might need to reinstitute one or more measures related to a specific part of the process for a short time. In most cases, all monitoring measures will be used during evaluation.

FIGURE 7-2. Level of Measurement Effort over Time

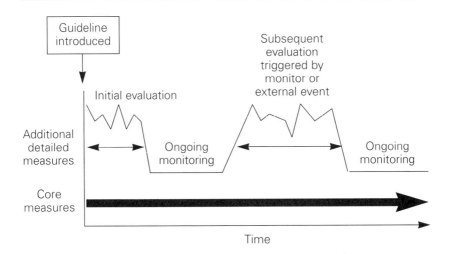

In considering how to select measures for monitoring and evaluation, we build on the input–process–outcome model in figure 7-1 by looking at three evaluation questions:

1. Is the guideline improving patient outcomes?
2. Is the guideline being used for the right patients?
3. Are the guideline recommendations being followed?

As we shall see below, considering the best way to address these questions might lead to some surprising choices of measures.

Is the Guideline Improving Patient Outcomes? This is the most important evaluation question for any guideline. Patient outcomes include clinical outcomes (mortality and morbidity) and functional status outcomes (activities of daily living, mobility, cognitive functioning). In addition, subjective measures of patient health status and patient satisfaction are now routinely collected in many health care organizations. The practice of including costs and resource utilization (length of stay, test ordering) in patient outcomes is controversial among clinicians, but it is indisputably a part of what drives many organizations to use guidelines in the first place.

To address the effects of a guideline on outcomes directly, one must compare the outcomes for patients managed using the guideline (appropriately adjusting for characteristics of the incoming patients) with the outcomes for patients managed without it. For many practice guidelines, the volume of cases seen and the resources available for long-term follow-up will make a true "clinical outcomes evaluation" difficult, if not impossible. Fortunately, a meaningful, practical evaluation can still be carried out by applying one simple principle: An evaluation can build on the results of published clinical studies without replicating them.

For example, when patients undergo hip replacement, deep vein thrombosis prophylaxis can reduce the postsurgical risk of embolism. However, for most delivery systems, the risk of embolism is small and the number of hip cases is not large enough to see a statistically significant reduction in this outcome. As long as guideline recommendations regarding deep vein thrombosis prophylaxis reflect the convincing evidence in the clinical literature, measuring compliance with the guideline is sufficient for a practical evaluation. We can invoke a previously established "chain of causes" to make the connection between the process of care and the desired patient outcome. Similarly, intermediate physiologic outcomes, such as the control of blood sugar levels in diabetics, can be linked through published studies to the patient outcomes we really care about: the risks of developing coronary disease or losing limbs.

A handful of major medical centers might have the talent and resources to turn every guideline evaluation into a publishable piece of clinical research. However, be warned that most published studies are supported by grants of several hundred thousand dollars from the National Institute of Health and take two or more years to complete. Insisting that every guideline evaluation follow the research model will limit an organization's capacity to improve patient outcomes. Most health care organizations can make major improvements in clinical quality by ensuring that already-proven "best practices" are consistently used in managing patient care. Evaluating the effects of such evidence-driven guidelines without attempting to replicate outcome studies is a much simpler process, one that can be completed in a matter of weeks or months rather than years. The following are key elements involved in an evaluation strategy to determine whether a guideline is improving patient outcomes.

Use existing measurement systems: Patient outcomes such as satisfaction and cost are highly dependent upon characteristics of a particular setting or delivery system. If these outcomes are critical, they might need to be measured directly, rather than by making inferences from published studies. Both the design of valid, reliable patient satisfaction surveys and the capturing of true costs are complex technical issues that go beyond the scope of this book. Fortunately, we can often harness existing information systems and ongoing patient satisfaction surveys to measure cost and satisfaction. In contrast, measuring clinical outcomes frequently requires a special evaluation system. While existing systems might have their shortcomings, the alternative (to ignore existing data and create parallel special studies) is wasteful and disruptive. For cost and satisfaction measurement, it is better to put the energy into improving what is already there! This element can be reduced to the following axiom and corollary:

- Axiom: The best monitoring systems are based on measurements that are seamlessly integrated into the existing work processes.
- Corollary: Save "special studies" for special situations (as during initial evaluation); adapt routine monitoring systems to meet routine needs.

Outcome measures must be related to severity of illness: To the extent that evaluation will rely on outcomes, the evaluation strategy must include a mechanism for case mix or severity adjustment. Patients with more advanced disease, with complicating comorbid conditions, or with other risk factors will generally have poorer outcomes than patients with less advanced disease, no comorbidities, and no risk factors.

Although everyone acknowledges the need for severity adjustment, clinicians are rarely satisfied with any particular adjustment method.

Since the introduction of diagnosis-related groups, a number of commercially available case mix and severity systems have been developed. Many of these rely on easily available clinical data—such as the International Classification of Diseases diagnosis and procedure codes—to assign the patients within a particular diagnosis-related group into one of four or five "severity strata."

Clinicians are rightfully wary of efforts to create generic severity scores that are applied over all possible medical and surgical conditions. Case mix or severity adjustments designed to explain differences in cost or length of stay are not necessarily appropriate when used to adjust mortality, morbidity, or functional status outcomes. Rather than relying on one "off-the-shelf" severity adjuster applied to every outcome for every guideline, organizations would do well to use clinically meaningful severity groups tailored to the outcomes and clinical conditions addressed by a particular guideline. Whatever method is used, concern lingers that differences in patient condition, rather than differences in process of care, explain differences in outcome.

Outcome measures do not explain why a guideline works: Even if outcomes are seen in theory as the "gold standard" for establishing the clinical effectiveness of a medical practice, the practical difficulties—adequate sample sizes, long lead times to observe some outcomes, concerns about severity adjustment—lead us to look beyond outcomes. There is a more compelling argument, however, for expanding our search for evaluation measures.

Outcome-based measures are really designed to answer the question: Is it working? This might seem to be sufficient for the long-term monitoring of an established guideline. However, as noted above, initial guideline evaluation and even long-term monitoring should also be designed to give insight into operational questions such as, "How does it work?" and "How does it fail?" Using only outcomes evaluation, it is difficult to understand the day-to-day operational implications of a guideline. If a guideline on administering prophylactic antibiotics makes no change in the postsurgical wound infection rate, is that because of the following?

- The guideline was not followed.
- The guideline recommendation was not different from pre-existing practice.
- The care recommended by the guideline made no difference.

Is the Guideline Being Used for the Right Patients? When guidelines are introduced, proponents are likely to be focused on getting providers to use the guideline, that is, to "comply" with its recommendations. In their enthusiasm, they might overlook the fact that a good guideline can make patient outcomes worse if it is used to manage the care of patients for whom it was never intended (for example, a guideline for routine ambulatory follow-up of patients with ischemic heart disease being applied to chest pain patients in an AIDS clinic). To determine whether the guideline is being used for the right patients, the following steps should be considered.

Measure which patients receive guideline care: Because guidelines might be implemented with varying degrees of formality and built-in system support, it might be difficult to tell which patients are being "managed on the guideline" and which are not. Some organizations expect all patients "on the guideline" to have a special documentation form in the chart. In other implementation settings, a physician can access a computer-based patient record that incorporates the guideline recommendations.[1] In other places, a guideline might have been distributed and discussed at grand rounds, and individual practitioners might or might not have changed their practices, but there is no special indication in the medical record that the guideline affected the care for this particular patient. Between these extremes, the indications that a patient is being managed "on the guideline" might be the use of special preprinted order forms, or of specially developed patient education materials.

Regardless of the formality with which the delivery system identifies and documents patients appropriate for a guideline, the evaluation system needs a set of measures that will permit the target patient population to be identified. Without such a denominator, it is not possible to say what fraction of the cases actually complied with guideline recommendations. In deciding how best to capture the number of cases that should be on the guideline, it is important to consider how patients might fail to be identified.

Consider why appropriate patients are not identified for guideline care: Patients might fail to be identified for guideline care for a number of reasons, including the following:

- They might be missed because they came by unorthodox routes. For example, a patient for amputation might usually be admitted through surgery, but might sometimes come through a medical service if other conditions actually initiated the hospital admission.
- They might develop symptoms during a stay that make them appropriate for a guideline that did not apply initially.
- It might be difficult in practice to make a timely decision to invoke a particular guideline. Key test results that will place a patient on or off a guideline might not be available at admission. For example, a patient arriving at the emergency room with chest pain and shortness of breath might be eligible for a pneumonia guideline or for a chest pain of ischemic origin guideline. Unless

these two guidelines share an initial "triage" section, it is possible that patients are identified as eligible for a guideline too late to follow key recommendations (such as delivering thrombolytic therapy to myocardial infarction patients within 30 minutes of admission to the emergency room).

Practical, usable guidelines must be constructed so that patients can be identified and managed in "real time." Guidelines with overlapping patient populations must be consistent and allow integration of care. These are guideline construction and implementation issues, but they directly impact the measurement and evaluation system.

For some guidelines, it is also important to identify patients who should not be on the guideline. If a test result is misinterpreted or a physical exam misses a key finding, a patient with a possible brain tumor might be treated using a depression guideline. In other cases, an initially suitable patient might have been improperly managed on a guideline even after exclusionary complications arose.

Use evaluation data to teach appropriate guideline use: Identifying cases where a guideline is being misapplied can guide improvements in the implementation process, especially during the initial evaluation. For example, conducting a grand rounds in which clinicians have a chance to run real cases through a guideline is a very effective teaching tool. Reviewing difficult cases in which the guideline seems to have been misapplied can make these sessions even more effective learning opportunities, and also lead to improvements in the wording or formatting of a guideline to reduce the chance of misinterpretation in the future.

In the early stages of implementing a guideline, another educational exercise is to conduct chart reviews to determine whether the right patients are being captured. However, chart review as a data collection strategy should never be viewed as more than a temporary measure. If a guideline is to become a permanent part of how an organization cares for a clinically meaningful group of patients, defined either by presenting symptoms or by a set of diagnostic criteria, then patients appropriate for guideline care must be identified routinely in "real time."

Are the Guideline Recommendations Being Followed? Many organizations are tempted to start and end with the question, "Are providers complying with the guideline?" The answer to this question is deceptively simple. Establishing a system to measure and monitor compliance is far from simple, as more than one organization has discovered. What exactly does it mean to "comply with a guideline" when the guideline might contain dozens of specific recommendations regarding tests, treatment, and follow-up care? If we try to measure compliance with every single guideline element, the burden of data collection can be overwhelming. The following elements must be considered when trying to address this question.

Defining compliance is not simple: Most guidelines are complex: an algorithmic format might have 10, 20, or 30 boxes; a single box might have a half dozen separate items. For any particular patient, defining compliance with even one item is not always obvious. Consider the case of a hypernatremic dehydration guideline calling for "administer[ing] 20 ml/kg 5% albumin IV immediately." Which of the following "comply" with the guideline recommendation?

- 19 ml/kg 5% albumin started 30 minutes after admission
- 20 ml/kg 5% albumin started 3 hours after admission
- 25 ml/kg 5% albumin started 15 minutes after admission and adjusted to 20 ml/kg 45 minutes later

The answer, of course, depends on how precisely the albumin dosage must be titrated to effect outcome and the meaning attached to "immediately."

Most diagnostic criteria or drug dosages are not as precise as guidelines make them appear. The cutoffs for establishing normal blood pressure versus hypertension, or borderline hypertension, are quite arbitrary given what we know about elevated blood pressure as a risk factor. Well-designed clinical trials might establish that a particular antibiotic dosage is effective against pneumococcus, without fully establishing the dose/response curve. In thrombolytic therapy or when using preoperative prophylactic antibiotics, timing is known to be important to the effectiveness of the drug, but attempts to establish precise time boundaries are doomed to be arbitrary. We know that the effectiveness of thrombolytic agents does not drop from fully effective to completely ineffective from one minute to the next.

Yet guidelines often include hard numbers as boundaries for deciding who should be considered hypertensive. Once that designation is made, a series of therapeutic recommendations will follow. The measure of compliance with a recommendation is almost always an all-or-nothing designation; that is, each case is either correctly managed (a value of 1) or incorrectly managed (a value of 0). In practice, we readily acknowledge what the scoring fails to recognize: that overlooking treatment for a "just-above-borderline" hypertensive patient is not as bad as failing to treat a patient with a blood pressure of 220/160. For a complex or time-dependent regimen, substituting a three-level score (fully, partially, or not compliant) for a 0–1 variable would better reflect reality and could easily be worth the extra complexity such scoring might add to the monitoring system.

Thus, in a situation such as this, the following axiom would hold true: The numerical precision of a guideline recommendation should not exceed that of the clinical studies on which it is based.

Degree of compliance required should be flexible: If measuring compliance with just one recommendation can be so technically challenging, attempting to monitor and evaluate compliance with every component of a guideline is sure to be a costly, frustrating, and counterproductive experience. When a guideline tries to dictate every detail of care, it will be rare to find a patient whose care rigidly complies with every single guideline recommendation. An overdefined compliance monitoring system quickly becomes a bad system for (mis)judging performance, rather than a good system for encouraging improvement. One way out is to invoke the Pareto principle, recognizing that a small fraction of the recommendations are truly critical in determining patient outcome. Thus, this axiom and corollary follow:

- Axiom: Not every guideline recommendation is equally important or equally evidence based.
- Corollary: Process measures should focus on the "vital few" recommendations—those grounded in the literature and critical to patient outcomes.

Limit the number of compliance measures: As we saw earlier, many problems that arise during the implementation of guidelines are rooted in the choice and construction of the guideline itself. Similarly, the key to establishing reasonable measurement and evaluation systems lies in the initial selection and tailoring of the guideline. If, after conscientiously weeding out the unsupported and inconsequential elements of a guideline, there are still more than four or five compliance measures, consider the possibility that the guideline itself is too complex.

Of course, some conditions do require complex guidelines, especially those aimed at standardizing the care of critically ill or severely compromised patients. The difficulty is that the human mind, even though capable of generating and codifying the guideline rules over a period of hours or days, might be unable to execute the rules reliably in the few minutes available for making decisions at the patient's bedside. For example, in the management of arterial oxygenation in the care of patients with adult respiratory distress syndrome in a pulmonary intensive care unit, the sheer volume of data on the patient's physiologic status is overwhelming, leading a physician to ignore all but three or four results (not necessarily the same three or four!) each time he or she reviews the patient's status. Not surprisingly, day-to-day decision making on the management of an adult respiratory distress syndrome patient is highly variable and not highly effective (commonly reported 30-day mortality rates of more than 85 percent).

For such a complex, data-rich set of decisions, a computerized protocol is a natural way to implement guideline-driven care. Once a draft guideline is generated and programmed, the problem of calibrating it presents an additional challenge. As with any guideline implementation, the question is how to interpret—and how to act on—cases in which its recommendations are inconsistent with the decisions made by the clinician in charge. In the case of a team at Latter Day Saints Hospital in Salt Lake City, the following "piloting" strategy was adopted prior to guideline implementation. During the pilot period, the computer protocol generated recommendations that physicians were allowed to override, and these were compared to the actual management decisions made for each patient. A team of experienced clinicians reviewed every case in which the computer recommendation and the physician action disagreed. For each disagreement, the team took one of the following three actions:

1. Affirm that the physician should have taken the action recommended by the protocol and give this feedback to the physician.
2. Affirm that the protocol was wrong and change it.
3. Affirm that the protocol was wrong and acknowledge that the situation was sufficiently unique and that the protocol should not be changed (remember, it is a feature of practical algorithms that they do not cover every situation).

The team then plotted the number of disagreements over time and concluded the pilot period when virtually all of them fell into the first or the third category. Interestingly, the pilot process, including feedback to the physicians, also greatly reduced the number of times the physicians incorrectly overrode the protocol recommendation. Once the computerized protocol was fully implemented, the 30-day survival rate among these patients increased dramatically from about 12 to 42 percent.[2]

STEPS FOR TAMING THE MEASUREMENT MONSTER

If the purpose of introducing clinical guidelines is to improve patient care, then measurement and evaluation are essential components. Ironically, the burden caused by measurement overdone and the dissension caused by measurement badly done can also be the undoing of a guideline. The measurement problem needs to be approached with the respect it deserves. The 10 steps below highlight important considerations you should make as you proceed:

1. Include measurement experts/map legacy system

When you form guideline teams, be sure to include access to technical experts in data collection, statistical analysis, and information systems. It is especially important that the guideline team knows about all the different legacy systems in the organization that are already collecting possibly relevant clinical and patient satisfaction data: financial systems; billing systems; Oryx systems; risk management systems; utilization review and case management systems; automated clinical record systems; and laboratory, pathology, and imaging department systems. A medical informatics specialist might be able to create an evaluation system by piecing together elements of these existing systems, minimizing the new data collection burden to the providers and bedside staff. (See table 7-1 for an overview of the role of experts and others in designing measurement systems.)

2. Think measurement early

The guideline team should initiate consideration of measurement and evaluation from the outset. Discussion of outcome measures can commence as soon as the topic of the guideline and the clinical population are defined. As guidelines are developed and reviewed, relevant data elements already captured in existing systems (see step 1) can be reviewed for validity and appropriateness. If measurement is considered early in the guideline development process, it might be possible to build into the guideline implementation unobtrusive ways to capture data not already available in legacy systems. In no circumstances should discussion of the problem of measurement and evaluation be left until after the guideline has been implemented!

3. Develop criteria for selecting measures

Develop a set of criteria for selecting the core monitoring measures. For all measures, the criteria should include the cost and feasibility of obtaining the data. For input measures, the criteria should weight the importance of and methods available for severity adjustment. The target population for a guideline needs to be identified in time to affect care, so the capture of input data necessary to identify guideline patients should be seamlessly integrated into the care. For process measures, selection criteria should focus attention on the relationship to outcome and the level of evidence. For outcome measures, end-result outcomes should be weighed against the value of proximate outcomes, physiologic markers, or process measures that have a demonstrated relationship to the desired end result.

TABLE 7-1. Measurement—Who's Involved?

Step in Measurement	Customers	Clinical Manager	Guidelines Team (Clinicians)	Data Analysts	Information Systems Analysts	Data Collectors
Define purpose of measurement	✓	✓	✓			
Identify key guideline components	✓		✓			
Define inputs	✓		✓	✓	✓	
Specify unit of analysis	✓		✓	✓	✓	
Identify data sources			✓	✓	✓	
Set measurement criteria			✓	✓	✓	
Document methods for data collection			✓	✓	✓	✓
Collect data and validate			✓	✓	✓	✓
Design report	✓		✓	✓		
Intercept findings	✓		✓			
Act on findings	✓	✓	✓			

4. Consider input, process, and outcome measures

Brainstorm a list of the possible core measures for each of the following categories:

- Input measures, including measures relating to diagnostic criteria, patient severity, and complexity
- Process measures relating to each guideline recommendation
- Outcome measures, including end-result measures, proximate measures, physiologic indicators predictive of outcome, and process measures predictive of outcome (there could be overlap with the process measures)

5. Choose practical care monitoring measures

Apply the selection criteria to establish a draft list of the core monitoring measures. Carefully consider the trade-off between the burden of collecting the measures and the value of the information gathered. Develop a detailed data collection plan for how each element will be collected, analyzed, reported, interpreted, and acted on. (See table 7-1.)

6. Choose temporary initial measures

Return to the brainstormed list from step 4 and identify additional measures that might be useful during the initial evaluation of the guideline and its implementation. Remember, these are not meant to become permanent fixtures in your measurement system!

7. Implement initial and ongoing measures

Implement the core measures for ongoing monitoring and the initial evaluation measures. Use the initial evaluation period as a time to validate, revise, and improve the ongoing monitoring system. Don't forget to ask for customer feedback about the reporting formats and ways in which core measures are summarized.

8. Meet weekly during initial evaluation

Meet weekly during the initial evaluation period to respond to what you are learning, to drop measures no longer needed, and to add new measures that will shed light on continuing problem areas.

9. End initial evaluation

When the team is satisfied with the level of performance based on the core indicators, declare that the initial evaluation period has ended and discontinue reporting of all but the core measures. Make sure the guideline tender agrees to review the ongoing monitoring reports and understands the criteria for activating a reevaluation of the guideline and its use. (See figure 7-2.)

10.   Continuously monitor core measures

Monitor the core measures and reactivate the team when a problem is identified, or when the guideline requires major revision and reassessment due to new scientific evidence or technical innovations in the way care is managed.

DISTINGUISH BETWEEN RESEARCH AND EVALUATION

As a final note of caution, the measurement and evaluation of guidelines will inevitably lead to tension regarding the reporting and interpretation of data. (It is important to remember that research refers to the assessment of guideline validity or efficacy, whereas evaluation refers to the assessment of guideline effectiveness.) The medical research model has profoundly shaped the thinking of most clinicians about how data "should" be presented and interpreted. Yet there is little reason to suppose that the same "level of evidence" should be required for two very different purposes:

1.   Establishing the value of a new procedure or drug in the first place (a medical research problem)
2.   Establishing the value of formally incorporating an already proven treatment into day-to-day practice

In courts of law, we recognize a standard of evidence required to convict a person accused of a crime with a consequence of depriving the person of liberty or even life: "beyond a reasonable doubt." A lesser standard of evidence is required to adjudicate a civil complaint where only money is involved: "the preponderance of the evidence." Scientific evidence, like its legal counterpart, builds on previous evidence and our assumptions about the world, pointing toward a conclusion with a greater or lesser degree of certainty. The very useful concept of testing the weight of scientific evidence with statistical tests has sometimes fostered the illusion that achieving "statistical significance" at the magic .05 level defines a "moment of truth." Prior to that moment nothing was known; after that moment all is known. In reality, the decision to "pay attention" to data if (and only if) a certain mathematical function falls below the number .05 is completely arbitrary. Had humans evolved with six fingers or four, our medical researchers and journal editors would, no doubt, be worshipping the .06 or .04 level of significance with the same (somewhat misplaced) enthusiasm.

Monitoring and evaluating the effects of guidelines on clinical care presents a practical rather than a research problem. We can solve that problem more effectively if we apply the same rigor of thought and method that we use to tackle research. However, we need to recognize that the stakes are different in designing systems to manage and improve day-to-day care in a single organization and conducting research on a new medical treatment that could affect the care of every patient on the planet. The management problem is better addressed if data are kept simple and accessible. Graphs and charts showing changes over time can be analyzed rigorously and at the same time allow everyone—patients, clinicians, managers—to see and understand the patterns at an intuitive level. (See figure 7-3 for example. Changes after the intervention in length of stay, deep vein thrombosis prophylaxis, and patient satisfaction are statistically significant.) That shared, intuitive grasp of what our data say is at least as important as the proper determination of a "p-value" in creating clinical teams capable of continuously improving the care rendered to patients.

Keys to Success

- Start with simple, evidence-based guidelines.
- Measure a handful of critical items well, rather than many items badly.
- Use existing data whenever possible.
- Focus measurement attention on the "vital few" recommendations that will impact outcomes.
- Focus measurement attention on the evidence-based elements of a guideline.
- Seek help from technical specialists in designing and implementing measures.

Operational Tips

- Treat guideline recommendations consistent with the degree of precision dictated by the clinical evidence.
- Sample when it makes sense—a reliable measure based on a sample of 25 cases is more meaningful than an erratic measure haphazardly collected on 500 cases.
- Don't be afraid to "turn off" or suppress detailed measures that are useful during the initial guideline evaluation, but are not critical for ongoing monitoring.
- Build on the clinical evidence—do not feel obligated to replicate the clinical studies on which the guideline is based.
- If precise, unvarying compliance with a guideline recommendations is important, build into the system of care a "foolproof" mechanism that always makes it happen.
- Find intuitive, informative ways to present data, using graphs of data over time rather than tables of numbers whenever possible (and it is always possible!).

FIGURE 7-3. Monitoring Care for Hip Replacement Patients

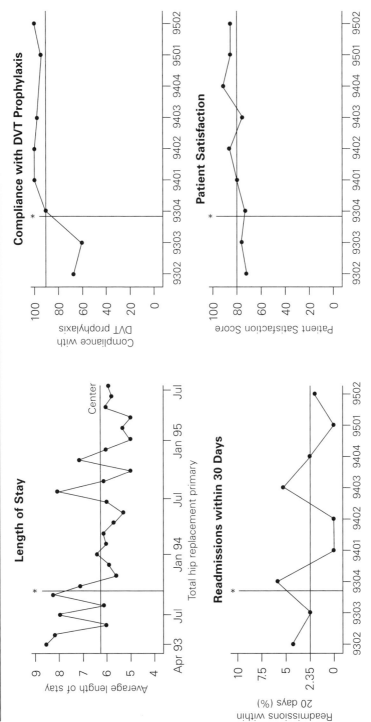

* = Guideline Introduced

137

References

1. D. L. Schriger, L. J. Baraff, W. H. Rogers, and S. Cretin, "Implementation of Clinical Guidelines Using a Computer Charting System: Effect on the Initial Care of Health Care Workers Exposed to Body Fluids," *JAMA* 278, no. 19 (1997): 1585-90.

2. A. H. Morris et al., "Randomized Clinical Trial of Pressure-Controlled Inverse Ratio Ventilation and Extracorporeal CO_2 Removal for Adult Respiratory Distress Syndrome," *Am. J. Resp. Crit. Care Med.* 149, no. 2, pt. 1 (1994): 295-305.

Implementing a Guideline Program: Two Case Studies

This chapter focuses on developing a guideline program. Two case studies—Kaiser Permanente, Georgia, a group-model health maintenance organization, and Children's Hospital, Boston, a tertiary care pediatric teaching hospital—are used to illustrate how two groups of people in different care settings and organizations succeeded in implementing a practice guideline program. The case studies are followed by comments that point out the strong similarities and particular differences between the implementation strategies described.

CASE 1. PLANNING AND RUNNING A CLINICAL PRACTICE GUIDELINES PROGRAM IN A GROUP-MODEL HEALTH MAINTENANCE ORGANIZATION: A PERSONAL ACCOUNT

by Dennis D. Tolsma, MPH, and Carole S. Gardner, MD

Kaiser Permanente, one of the nation's largest health maintenance organizations, has been in existence for more than 50 years. Long-established Kaiser Permanente plans have led the creation of formal guideline programs. However, the Kaiser Permanente Medical Care Program in Georgia is one of the newer plans and had only a handful of protocols in place prior to 1994. That year, Kaiser Permanente, Georgia, launched a major program to develop clinical practice guidelines. Despite the program's lack of experience, the initial clinical teams identified 117 clinical conditions meriting clinical practice guidelines. The impetus to undertake so extensive a task came from the following sources:

- Lack of consistency in referrals to specialists: Provider support for guidelines began to emerge as the medical group became aware how much its own practice habits influenced referrals.
- Growing competition in the Atlanta marketplace, with both pressures on rates and demands by buyers to demonstrate efficient, high-quality care.
- A decision to seek and win accreditation by the National Committee on Quality Assurance.
- Top management support, as evidenced by the appointment of Bruce Perry, MD, MPH, as Associate Medical Director for Clinical Affairs. Perry had had extensive experience in the Group Health Cooperative of Puget Sound, an early leader in the field of clinical practice guidelines known for applying guidelines in its innovative prevention and clinical road map programs.[1]

Planning the Clinical Practice Guideline Program

Perry brought with him a vision of a clinical improvement program that placed in one organization, a new Division of Clinical Affairs, an array of resources aimed at continuous quality improvement of care. Perry defined the scope of the division as "everything that isn't operations," and explicitly included one unit, the Clinical Practice Analysis and Support Department, to coordinate a comprehensive program of clinical practice guideline development and implementation. His template for quality included six functions that are described below under the titles of the new departments:

1. Quality Resource Management

Quality Resource Management provides the essential medical management coordination functions of any managed care organization—utilization management, case management across the continuum, support to the hospital rounding teams, alternate products management (for example, network, point of service), and referral management.

2. Risk Management

This department pursues an active program of acquisition of risk information, consultation, oversight, physician training, benefits coordination and exception, etc.

3. Health Information Management

The primary mission of this unit is defining, documenting, and implementing systems that help to ensure that appropriate and accurate clinical information is complete and available when needed. Special emphasis has been placed on a major effort to implement an electronic medical record to be utilized by the Georgia market area clinical staff to enhance the delivery of quality patient care.

4.   Quality Assessment, Improvement, and Reporting

Quality Assessment, Improvement, and Reporting has three primary responsibilities: (1) leadership of quality improvement strategies and initiatives, (2) oversight of professional peer review, and (3) oversight of professional credentialing and recredentialing. Within a framework called the quality imperative, strategies included maintaining current full, three-year National Committee on Quality Assurance accreditation, attaining market-best Health Plan Employer Data & Information Set (HEDIS) performance, assisting the national Kaiser Permanente program in the sharing of best clinical practices, utilizing monthly meetings of the Quality Forum to facilitate needed strategic change, developing and implementing disease state management programs, and profiling the performance of internal and network providers as a tool for clinical practice improvement.

5.   Prevention, Health Promotion, and Research

This department was created to offer a comprehensive health education and workplace health promotion program, to design and deliver new products and system supports (such as prevention reminder systems, immunization outreach programs, and office-based smoking cessation services), to create evidence-based prevention guidelines for clinical preventive services, and to inaugurate a research program capable of competing for externally funded clinical and health services research studies.

6.   Clinical Practice Analysis and Support

This department is involved in the coordination of clinical practice guidelines in general and carries out a program of development of the majority of the clinical practice guidelines at Kaiser Permanente, Georgia. Clinical Practice Analysis and Support provides support with writing, editing, data abstraction and analysis, and group facilitation. It also promotes strategies to disseminate and use guidelines through assistance to the service and specialty chiefs charged with this accountability, to define measures by which to monitor and feed back use of guidelines, and to conduct outcome studies. More recently, Clinical Practice Analysis and Support became the project lead for the Kaiser Permanente, Georgia, Diabetes Disease State Management Program and the Coordinated Asthma Management Program.

An important feature of the division is the partnership of departmental leaders—each has a clinical chief (who also practices in primary care) and a full-time director, who jointly plan and carry out the departmental mission. While Perry was assembling this leadership team, he personally led the initial development of "edition one" of what were then called "Referral Guidelines."

Developing the Initial Clinical Practice Guidelines

The Kaiser Permanente, Georgia, approach to guidelines at the outset was consciously based on a "medical consensus" strategy. This was due, in part, to the need to bring the medical group into guidelines step-by-step and to accommodate initial wariness about intrusion into medical practice preferences. It was also simply a pragmatic response to the need to get something in place rapidly. The development teams' meetings were sometimes stormy and sometimes able to produce only rudimentary guidance. Yet, in a surprisingly short period of time, a significant array of guidelines were distributed to the primary care providers and specialists of Kaiser Permanente, Georgia. Late in the process, Perry recruited the authors and turned over the Clinical Practice Analysis and Support mission to them with the familiar Nike charge, "Just Do It."

Dr. Gardner came to Kaiser Permanente, Georgia, from practice in general internal medicine and geriatrics. Named as Chief of Clinical Practice Analysis and Support for the medical group, she brought a background in academic medicine at the University of Kentucky and the Veterans Administration. Her partner, Mr. Tolsma, was appointed Director of Prevention and Practice Analysis and was responsible for prevention initiatives, practice guidelines and studies, and disease state management. He came to Kaiser Permanente, Georgia, with a public health background, having served as Director of the Center for Health Promotion and Education and later as Associate Director for Public Health Practice at the Centers for Disease Control and Prevention, where he directed programs that combined technology transfer and applied research missions. Each brought a strong interdisciplinary background to the Division.

The first step was to form teams for guideline development. A later step, after the first set of guidelines had been developed, was to shift guideline development emphasis to evidence-based approaches.

Forming Guideline Teams/Development Process   Each guideline team was composed of a relevant specialist, several primary care providers, and a representative from pharmacy. Occasionally, other subject matter experts (for example, registered dietitians) are added if the topic suggests a need. Clinical Practice Analysis and Support staff, which include a guidelines development coordinator, a clinical process consultant, and a research associate, assist each team in several ways, including the following:

- Identifying and distributing "seed guidelines," typically guidelines prepared in other Kaiser Permanente medical care programs
- Performing literature searches and preparing evidence tables
- Taking minutes and drafting or redrafting initial guideline text for team review (much of the text is typically produced by the staff based on notes, followed by review and editing by the teams)
- Occasionally generating internal data on referrals or encounters to help teams assess current practice patterns

Typically, two formal meetings are convened and facilitated by Clinical Practice Analysis and Support, with team members assigned prework and follow-up between meetings. Participants are awarded continuing medical education credits based on the literature research and formal presentations made at these sessions. Most important, for the second edition, which added an additional 87 referral guidelines and a full revision of the entire set a year later, Clinical Practice Analysis and Support endeavored to gradually shift the approach from "consensus based" to "evidence based."

Shifting to Emphasize Evidence Base of Guidelines This philosophic change acknowledges that wide practice variation exists in any medical group and that "beliefs," preferences, past experience, and even the most astute clinical impressions offer no guarantee that such guidance will produce the best, or even good, clinical practices. At Kaiser Permanente, Georgia, the development of practice guidelines accepts that there might be no compelling evidence to determine choices about some clinical circumstances, but that there is a hierarchy of approaches for applying increasingly rigorous judgments in developing clinical practice guidelines. David Eddy has suggested that these can be arrayed under the headings "global subjective judgment," "evidence based," "outcomes based," and "preference based."[2] He notes that evidence-based approaches have the advantage of consciously anchoring a policy, not to opinions, but to experimental evidence. Going beyond this to estimating the magnitude of benefits and harms (outcomes based) and to including patient preferences for outcomes (preference based) was beyond the scope of data, human resources, and time at Kaiser Permanente, Georgia, at that point.

However, Clinical Practice Analysis and Support and the department chiefs made a conscious decision to push the teams toward evidence-based approaches. In parallel, an interdisciplinary prevention committee assembled guideline teams of practitioners from medicine, pediatrics, and obstetrics-gynecology, with the same charge. Both sets of products—

prevention and referral guidelines—were distributed to the medical group primary care providers in the second half of 1995.

Introducing the Guidelines to the Clinicians

At that point, the Kaiser Permanente, Georgia, program of provider-developed guidelines had fully met the National Committee on Quality Assurance standards, and Kaiser Permanente, Georgia, received its full three-year National Committee on Quality Assurance accreditation in 1995. In introducing the guidelines to their clinical colleagues, Perry and the Clinical Practice Analysis and Support team understood that the information was still basic and often less specific than many physicians desired; however, guidelines are intended simply as guides. As Perry put it, they were intended to fit 95 percent of the clinical conditions encountered 95 percent of the time, but not to substitute for the "activated frontal lobes of the clinician." Moreover, they were still geared toward providing criteria for referral to specialists.

As the guideline development strategy at Kaiser Permanente, Georgia, evolved, Clinical Practice Analysis and Support decided to modify its guidelines approach toward a diagnosis-driven format. The team also collected data from primary care practitioners and from specialists to whom patients were referred, in an effort to understand ways in which to improve guidelines implementation and enhance clinician acceptance and use of the clinical practice guideline. Clinical Practice Analysis and Support also began to test ways in which to provide data feedback to primary care providers regarding practice patterns under the guidelines.

Referral or Specialty-Oriented Guidelines versus Diagnosis or Problem-Oriented Guidelines In concept, referral guidelines are just clinical practice guidelines in a different format. However, rather than being driven by diagnosis, they were organized around specialty departments. The clinician began with the notion of what specialty this problem might belong to if referred, rather than the clinical diagnosis suspected. This had the initial advantage of focusing clinical attention on appropriate referring practices, but strained clinical logic and sometimes evoked confusion and duplication. For example, "shoulder pain" might be found under orthopedics, but also under physical therapy, and even under rheumatology. Moreover, learnings from a referral monitoring pilot project and from a physician survey suggested that greater benefits could be gained from shifting to a diagnosis-driven framework while retaining and rationalizing the criteria for referral within a given diagnosis. Thus, in formulating its 1996–97 guidelines plan, Clinical Practice Analysis and

Support set out to issue a comprehensive clinical practice guideline document that incorporated a complete revision and reframing of the clinical practice guideline. The timetable was based on the 1996 National Committee on Quality Assurance standard for practice guidelines, which requires that clinical practice guidelines should be revised no less frequently than every two years.

Two Studies on Monitoring Provider Satisfaction with Guidelines

To better understand the reception and impact of practice guidelines at Kaiser Permanente, Georgia, Clinical Practice Analysis and Support undertook two studies. The first study was to design, with the assistance of a Centers for Disease Control and Prevention analyst detailed to work with Clinical Practice Analysis and Support on a personnel exchange, a 1996 survey of the Kaiser Permanente, Georgia, practitioner attitudes and beliefs about clinical practice guidelines and views about how to make them more useful. With permission of the managing physician, the questionnaire was administered in person at the regular provider meeting of each of the nine Kaiser Permanente, Georgia, medical centers, in order to ensure an acceptable response rate. A list of providers who did not attend the meeting was used to mail questionnaires, and additional responses were obtained in this way. Although administered largely in person, the survey itself was anonymous, to elicit candor. The design team had the advantage of a useful set of attitudinal questions developed by S. R. Tunis, R. S. A. Hayward, and M. C. Wilson. These questions had been administered to a population consisting largely of physicians in private practice and academic medicine.[3]

Results of the the Kaiser Permanente, Georgia, survey were encouraging.[4] Physicians indicated that they used the guidelines at least some of the time, for some diagnoses. In virtually every category of attitudinal response, the Kaiser Permanente, Georgia, providers were more receptive to guidelines than those surveyed by Tunis. They were also less likely to believe that guidelines were cookbook medicine or were likely to be used punitively. Finally, a large majority of the Kaiser Permanente, Georgia, respondents agreed with an overall question about whether guidelines should be used by the Kaiser Permanente, Georgia, practitioners. While not assured that guidelines were actually being used, the Clinical Practice Analysis and Support team concluded from these data that their health maintenance organization setting offered a receptive climate and positive support for the two-year-old program of clinical practice guideline development and implementation.

A second pilot project was undertaken in late 1995 and continued through early 1996. It was intended to redesign the referral management process and to add a measurement process. As indicated above, increasing the appropriateness of specialist referrals was a high priority and was also an important consideration of the primary care reengineering effort being pilot tested at the same time. The project team was composed of Clinical Practice Analysis and Support and other stakeholders. Our intent was to track the volume of referrals by diagnosis, to identify whether they were made under 1 of the 220 referral guidelines, and, if they were, to test whether they were consistent with the guideline. The "gold standard" was whether the receiving specialist concurred with the indication by the primary care provider that the referral was consistent with the guideline. (The primary care provider was also given the option to indicate other reasons for referring, such as clinical judgment of necessity.) A feature of the pilot measurement system was a text field called "educational exchange." The instructions suggested that the specialist offer "educational guidance on additional things that could be done in primary care when this clinical condition is encountered" and that the form be returned to the primary care provider as a private communication. Although not always used by the specialist, many primary care providers found the educational exchange feature to be a valuable feedback tool and a relatively neutral and nonthreatening way to learn how to manage care in specific referral decisions.

It is not the purpose of this chapter to describe primary care provider and specialist referral issues. Suffice it to say, the Clinical Practice Analysis and Support team learned a great deal about primary care provider–specialist relationships and the difficulty of sustaining complex process flows in busy practices. The pilot was ultimately not extended throughout the medical centers for unrelated reasons—an impending shift in computer platforms and development of a new claims and referral management system. Nevertheless, the authors strongly believe that both development and implementation of guidelines programs will be well served by monitoring systems that include the capability to track appropriateness as a fundamental aspect of integrating primary and specialty care.

Use of Appropriateness Data for Feedback to Providers Data on appropriateness would have many uses. For guidelines developers, those clinical practice guidelines that consistently yield referrals deemed inconsistent with the guidelines are probably inferior or unclear products and should be withdrawn and revised. Aggregation and dissemination of these data to providers in the form of peer comparison feedback would enable individual providers to recognize where their practice patterns are out of line with their peers; and, when the feedback is provided unblinded, it gives them an opportunity to seek out respected colleagues to learn how to modify practice habits. In our medical groups, service chiefs are responsible for overseeing the content and quality of care. Aggregated data permit them to identify the specific diagnostic areas where one or several primary care providers could benefit from continuing medical education and thus to better target scarce educational time and resources. The Clinical Practice Analysis and Support team plans to reintroduce this monitoring approach when the systems and referral management processes exist to support it.

Data feedback to clinicians regarding use of guidelines is also a primary component of disease state management programs. Kaiser Permanente, Georgia, tracks a number of data items relevant to diabetes and asthma guidelines, and distributes to primary care providers quarterly reports of panel-specific data. The metrics tracked are both intermediate outcomes (for example, for diabetes, the percent of patients in glycemic control) and procedures (for example, the percent of patients receiving two or more hemoglobin A1c blood tests in the past 12 months). These data help primary care providers to identify and address care needs at both the individual patient and whole population levels.

Disseminating the Revised Guidelines

Clinical Practice Analysis and Support introduced the comprehensively revised and reformatted guidelines in July 1997. Feedback from the provider survey suggested that one problem was accessibility in the modules of the referral guidelines. Originally disseminated in a bulky three-ring binder format, the new clinical practice guidelines were reformatted to expedite their use, with several additional new features, including the following:

- The clinical practice guidelines are bound in a pocketbook format, sized to fit in the pocket of a medical coat.
- All diagnoses are now listed in alphabetical order, rather than subindexed by specialty.
- All clinical practice guidelines were also made available to primary care providers in early 1998 in the Kaiser Permanente, Georgia, intranet—that is, in hypertext format accessible through the intranet browser.
- Each clinical practice guideline is formatted vertically to flow logically from "suggested evaluation" to "treatment options" to "referral criteria."
- In development work for launching an on-line medical record in 1999, the Clinical Practice Analysis and Support chief collaborated with health informatics staff in developing a series of "prompts" for all conditions for which clinical practice guidelines referral criteria exist. A Referral Order Management System is an initial module in the electronic record system. The prompts are in the form of questions referenced to specific clinical practice

guidelines, which the clinician triggers while starting a computer-based referral order for a specific diagnosis.

- The publication is a comprehensive compilation of the Kaiser Permanente, Georgia, guidelines. In addition to the text of all clinical practice guidelines, it contains the prevention guidelines; a detailed imaging guideline; the text and care paths of the guideline prepared for the Diabetes Disease State Management Program; and cross-references to the therapy guidelines prepared by the Pharmacy and Therapeutics Committee for acid peptic disorders, hypertension, and dyslipidemia.
- Each clinical practice guideline specifies the health education materials and/or patient education classes considered appropriate for the specified conditions (all educational materials were reviewed by both a clinician and a health educator to ensure that they supported and were consistent with the clinical practice guideline).

Lessons Learned

There are a number of implementation strategies identified in the medical literature.[5] Clinical Practice Analysis and Support and other stakeholders in the clinical practice guideline process have employed several of these. All groups contemplating a guideline process should bear in mind several lessons from this experience.

First, although there might be skepticism about whether guidelines really matter, the clinical practice guideline team will almost immediately receive a growing volume of requests in the form of "we need a guideline for this topic and we need it quick." It is essential to find some formal or informal structure that can help set priorities among these many competing needs.

Second, from the outset, clinical practice guideline development should consciously include attention to the dissemination strategies by which the clinical practice guideline will be rolled out to the clinicians. We learned that much time is lost searching for mechanisms once the publication is in hand. Formal continuing medical education, while perhaps the easiest or most obvious choice, might not be the right one.

Third, each implementation strategy has a cost, and not all strategies are cost-effective in all circumstances. The cost is more than the direct expense of organizing the intervention; physician release time is a precious resource in most health maintenance organizations today. Be prudent and realistic in making choices among strategies.

Fourth, the measurements and data capture needed to monitor clinical practice guideline use and impact should also be part of the process at the outset rather than created at the end. Ideally, even before guidelines are written, the authors of guidelines themselves should be asked to identify what will be different if practice variation is reduced and quality of care is improved, and what metric will track any change.[6] In its current clinical practice guideline, Kaiser Permanente, Georgia, has only a few such measures defined *a priori*. However, in the Disease State Management Program, a range of specific outcomes and data systems needed to track them were created in conjunction with the guideline and the process improvement efforts. The Clinical Practice Analysis and Support team sees this as the strategy of choice for future guideline development efforts.

Fifth, the ideal for clinical practice guidelines is to embed them in the clinical practice routine, and there are real advantages to practicing in an integrated delivery system such as our group-model health maintenance organization. In the current marketplace reality, however, virtually all managed care organizations are or are becoming mixed models. Introducing the clinical practice guideline program into other products, such as independent practice association networks, is even more complicated and will likely require different strategies than those we have tried.

Sixth, for a variety of reasons, ranging from medical group buy-in to compliance with National Committee on Quality Assurance standards, providers must be actively involved in the clinical practice guideline effort. However, they must be supported by talented staff (though it need not be a large infrastructure). Clinical Practice Analysis and Support is fortunate to have a team that is well organized and versatile, with members who have skills in writing, editing, data abstraction and analysis, and group facilitation. We also see both our providers and our members as customers of the ultimate products of the effort. It would be very difficult to succeed without these types of resources supporting the guidelines effort.

Summary

Much of this account has addressed the topic of development of practice guidelines. There is little doubt that this activity has become very important as one of the hallmarks of true managed care, with its focus on reducing practice variation and continuous quality improvement. There is also little doubt that just developing guidelines alone will have marginal effect. Clinical Practice Analysis and Support has evolved its mission over the past year. While still the leader in clinical practice guideline development, Clinical Practice Analysis and Support now increasingly views its role as including clinical practice guideline implementation and clinical practice guideline monitoring. Both are challenges, at Kaiser Permanente, Georgia, and any other medical group.

Bruce Perry became medical director of the Kaiser Permanente Medical Care Program in Georgia in 1996, but remains the executive sponsor of guidelines implementation, along with his senior medical staff. Kaiser Permanente, Georgia, has moved from having no formal guidelines program to having a comprehensive guideline development effort in less than three years. We still recognize weaknesses in the clinical practice guidelines themselves, and still see clinical topics that merit new clinical practice guidelines. We remain acutely aware that use of the clinical practice guidelines in daily care delivery is less widespread and assiduous than we would like. We have only begun to find ways to build ongoing monitoring and feedback systems to track use of guidelines and their effect on quality of care. Finally, we are keenly aware that the proof of the pudding is in the eating—that we need to undertake outcome studies to demonstrate guideline impact and redirect resources toward achieving improved outcomes. Progress in all of these aims forms the clinical practice guideline agenda for Kaiser Permanente, Georgia, over the next three years.

References and Notes

1. J. F. Beekman, "Will Clinicians Accept Practice Guidelines?" *Health Maintenance Organization Practice* 5, no. 3 (1991): 109-11.

2. D. M. Eddy, *A Manual for Assessing Health Practices and Designing Health Practice Policies: The Explicit Approach* (Philadelphia: American College of Physicians, 1992).

3. S. R. Tunis, R. S. A. Hayward, M. C. Wilson et al., "Internists' Attitudes about Clinical Practice Guidelines," *Ann. Intern. Med.* 120 (1994): 257-63.

4. C. S. Gardner, D. Guthrie, and C. Swofford, "Use of and Attitudes toward Clinical Practice Guidelines," Southern Regional Meeting of the Society of General Internal Medicine, New Orleans, LA, Feb. 6, 1997.

5. M. R. Handley, M. E. Stuart, H. L. Kirz, "Effective Implementation of Clinical Practice Guidelines," *Health Maintenance Organization Practice* 8, no. 2 (1994).

6. B. C. James, "Good Enough? Standards and Measurement in Continuous Quality Improvement," in *Bridging the Gap between Theory and Practice* (Chicago: Hospital Research and Education Trust [American Hospital Association], 1992).

CASE 2. ESTABLISHING AND RUNNING A CLINICAL PRACTICE GUIDELINE PROGRAM AT CHILDREN'S HOSPITAL, BOSTON

by Rita Gibes Grossman, RN, MSc; Charles Homer, MD, MPH; and Donald A. Goldmann, MD

Children's Hospital, Boston, launched a formal clinical practice guideline program in 1993 in response to market demands for high-quality care at a competitive price. The hospital's definition of a clinical practice guideline is as follows: A clinical practice guideline is a systematically developed, evidence- and consensus-based, multidisciplinary plan of care for a specific patient population that serves as a guide for clinical decision making and as a method to ensure that all aspects of the care process are carried out in a timely fashion to best meet the patients' needs. This definition emphasizes the evidence- and consensus-based attributes of guidelines as defined by the Institute of Medicine[1] and the efficiency characteristics associated with critical pathways, which seek to standardize care and ensure that the critical steps in providing care are done in a timely fashion.[2]

Our goals in establishing clinical practice guidelines were to improve or maintain high-quality care while becoming more efficient, primarily by reducing waste and unnecessary variation in practice. This case study discusses these key concepts and the practical aspects of implementing clinical practice guidelines in a large, tertiary care pediatric teaching hospital.

Initiating the Clinical Practice Guideline Program

Prior to the spring of 1993, three nearly simultaneous events led to the creation of the Children's Hospital, Boston, Clinical Practice Guideline Program.

First, the Cardiovascular Program, a self-contained, comprehensive cardiac care program within Children's Hospital, Boston, implemented a critical pathway program.[3] The implementation of its first critical pathway for secundum-type atrial septal defect reduced the average length of stay by 0.6 of a day and decreased associated laboratory costs by 14.6 percent.[4]

Second, a group of clinicians driven by concerns about the variations in the quality of care developed a clinical practice guideline for patients with pelvic inflammatory disease. The pelvic inflammatory disease guideline clarified the process of care for patient teaching, screening for sexually transmitted diseases, diagnostic testing, and treatment. The roles of adolescent medicine, gynecology, surgery, nursing, and social work were spelled out. Not only were improvements in patient teaching and sexually transmitted disease screening documented, but reductions in length of stay (25 percent) and charges (10 percent) were achieved.[5]

Third, Children's Hospital, Boston, became the primary pediatric hospital for a large health maintenance organization, the Harvard Community Health Plan (HCHP).[6] This health maintenance organization contributed guideline expertise as well as a negotiated expectation that clinical practice guidelines would be part of clinical improvement activities at Children's Hospital, Boston. The encouraging results of the cardiovascular critical pathways and the pelvic inflammatory disease guideline, coupled with the HCHP partnership agreement, catalyzed the development of a formal hospitalwide program to support clinical practice guideline activity.

The program was designed in eight months by a multidisciplinary committee, the Clinical Practice Guideline Steering Committee. It was cochaired by the medical director of quality improvement and by a clinical nurse specialist who was the acting director of the multidisciplinary intensive care unit at that time. They were chosen to lead this effort based on their clinical credibility and their demonstrated leadership ability. A nurse clinical specialist with management experience and a masters in health policy and management was chosen to design and direct the program, with direction from the Clinical Practice Guideline Steering Committee.

Building on the experience of the cardiovascular program and of the pelvic inflammatory disease clinicians, the Clinical Practice Guideline Steering Committee developed the following:

- The clinical practice guideline program mission and vision, and the clinical practice guideline topic selection criteria (see exhibit 8-1 for the committee's mission statement)
- A carefully conceived, detailed, annotated process for clinical practice guideline development based on the Institute of Medicine recommendations (see exhibit 8-2)[7]
- Recommendations for the format of clinical practice guideline clinical documents
- Institutional activities to enhance clinical practice guideline acceptance

While writing the mission and vision, program leadership foresaw the potential for conflict between the goals of improving patient care quality and reducing costs. Improving quality was the cornerstone of our vision statement and was the primary objective for clinicians, while the administration was concerned with costs. The Clinical Practice Guideline Program leaders and hospital administration agreed that improving the quality of care might not always have an immediate, measurable impact on cost.

EXHIBIT 8-1. Clinical Practice Guidelines Steering Committee: Vision/Mission Statement

---

VISION STATEMENT

To promote optimal patient[1] outcomes[2] by providing the highest quality of care through a process that is:

- Individualized[3]
- Appropriate[4]
- Valid[5]
- Predictable[6]
- Able to be evaluated
- Cost effective[7]
- Of the greatest possible value to the community.

MISSION STATEMENT

The Clinical Practice Guideline Steering Committee (CPGSC) has been charged by the Continuous Improvement Committee to lead the development of an institutional framework and collaborative process for the implementation of Clinical Practice Guidelines (CPGs). The CPG Steering Committee will:

- Identify criteria[8] for determining which care processes will be targeted for CPG development.
- Develop standards[9] and criteria for the process of CPG development, implementation and evaluation. Evaluation will be defined in terms of process, outcomes[2], cost and resource utilization.
- Develop standards and criteria for the timely revision and updating of CPGs.
- Support the identification of opportunities for research.
- Promote clinician education through the CPG process.

The CPG Steering Committee is accountable to the Medical Staff Quality Improvement Committee, collaborates with other committees and supports the overall strategic plan of Children's Hospital.

DEFINITION OF TERMS

1. **Patient.** The individual patient and the family/significant others who are part of a community.

2. **Outcomes.** Reflect the integration of such variables as physiologic, functional status, quality of life, access, cost-effectiveness, value and patient satisfaction.

3. **Individualized.** The supremacy of the unique needs of the patient (e.g. social, developmental, etc.) is recognized over the guidelines which are designed for the general population.

4. **Appropriate.** Care for which the expected health benefits exceed expected health risks by a sufficiently wide margin so that the care is worth delivering.

(Continued on next page)

EXHIBIT 8-1. (Continued)

5. **Valid.** Guidelines and/or algorithms that are "evidence based."

6. **Predictable.** The patient care process will be similar for patients with similar illnesses.

7. **Cost Effective**. Recognizes the need to provide the highest quality of care using available resources within the system.

8. **Criteria.** Elements that are able to be measured to specify desired characteristics of outcome, process or structure.

9. **Standards.** The predetermined "targets" or range of values by which criteria or variables will be measured.

Criteria for CPG Process Selection

The following criteria have been prepared to serve as guidelines for selecting the target processes for clinical practice guideline development.

1. Data and clinician judgment indicate an opportunity to **improve the quality of care.**

2. **High volume** patient population where an improved process would yield a net benefit for the individual patient as well as for the entire population. There should be enough patient volume to capture variability and measure impact of changes.

3. **Variation in practice patterns** exist within the organization as well as when compared to other pediatric health care organizations in:
   - LOS
   - utilization (e.g. tests, medications, services, etc.) or
   - lack of consensus on "best" process of care.

4. Resource utilization and case mix data indicate an **opportunity to reduce costs** without negatively affecting the quality of care.

5. Opportunity to evaluate a **new method or technology** prior to its integration into clinical practice.

6. Improve the use of an existing application or technology.

The following issues should also be considered:
- Opportunity to link providers/disciplines/departments.
- Clinician interest.
- Patient oriented and population directed.
- Feasible topic (e.g. data available; realizable goal).
- Measurable endpoints: Able to evaluate impact of CPG on practice?
- Is volume sufficient to allow analysis of process and variance?
- Is this an opportunity to reduce costs while maintaining or improving quality?

EXHIBIT 8-2. Overview of Clinical Practice Guidelines Process

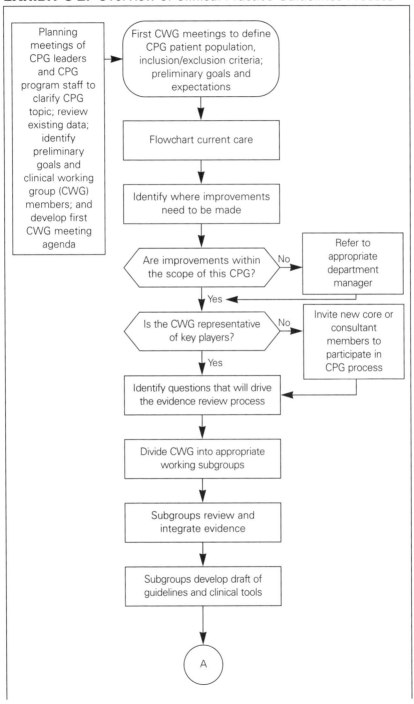

(Continued on next page)

EXHIBIT 8-2. (Continued)

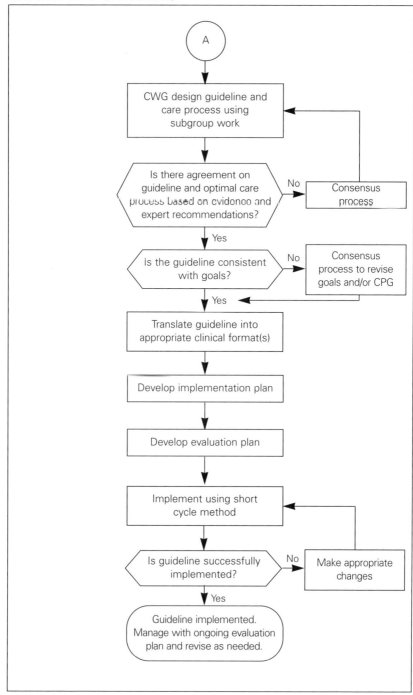

Developing the Clinical Practice Guideline Program

Clinical Practice Guideline Program staff included a program director (0.6 full-time equivalent); coordinators who provide executive level support for development, implementation, and evaluation (1.2 full time equivalent); an analyst (0.2 full-time equivalent); secretarial support (0.2 full time equivalent); and a designated clinical practice guideline consultant from the finance department. The program is administratively based in the Quality Improvement Department and also works closely with the Clinical Effectiveness Program, a research and training program in pediatric health services research.

In January 1994, clinical practice guideline development began for four diagnoses. Topics were chosen with motivated, self-recruited leaders. Since that time, 17 guidelines have been completed and four more are in early phases of development (see exhibit 8-3).

EXHIBIT 8-3. List of Operational Guidelines

CPG	Principal Department *(In collaboration with Nursing and other departments)*
Asthma - Inpatient	Medicine
Asthma - Emergency	Emergency Medicine
Bronchiolitis	Medicine
Cystic Fibrosis	Medicine
Diabetes (newly diagnosed)	Medicine
Fever & Neutropenia	Oncology
Gastroenteritis	Medicine/Gastroenterology
Hyperbilirubinemia	Newborn Medicine
Intravenous Immunoglobulin	Medicine
Osteomyelitis	Orthopedic Surgery
Pleural Effusion	Medicine/Emergency Medicine
Pelvic Inflammatory Disease	Medicine
Ruptured Appendectomy	General Surgery
Septic Arthritis	Orthopedic Surgery

Suicidality
    Emergency
    Medical Inpatient
    Psychiatric Inpatient
	Psychiatry

Total Parenteral Nutrition	Gastroenterology
Urinary Tract Infection (< two years of age)	Medicine
Ventriculo-peritoneal Shunt	Neurosurgery

The Clinical Practice Guideline Program provides expert consultation to clinicians through each phase of clinical practice guideline development, implementation, and evaluation.

Clinical Practice Guideline Development In terms of development, Clinical Practice Guideline Program staff members work closely with the clinical practice guideline coleaders in order to do the following:

- To identify appropriate topics for clinical practice guideline work
- To work with the finance department to obtain case-mix data and resource utilization data
- To select and organize the clinical working group that will develop and implement the clinical practice guideline
- To facilitate clinical working group meetings and meetings of the clinical practice guideline coleaders
- To support the scheduling and agenda planning for these meetings
- To provide a succinct, immediate written summary of each meeting, accompanied by a "to do" list noting the responsible person for each item on the list

Clinical Practice Guideline Implementation In terms of implementation, program staff members work with the coleaders in order to do the following:

- To create and refine clinical practice guideline documents through production and subsequent revisions
- To develop an implementation plan and support deployment activities.

Clinical Practice Guideline Evaluation In terms of evaluation, the program staff members work with coleaders in order to do the following:

- To develop an evaluation plan, define process and outcome measures, and identify data elements and methods needed to acquire data
- To provide support for analysis and reporting of data to clinical working group

Incorporating the Elements into the Clinical Practice Guideline Process at Children's Hospital, Boston

Following are some of the elements that the clinical practice guideline designers took into consideration when developing their program at Children's Hospital, Boston.

Involvement of the Residents Because Children's Hospital, Boston, is a tertiary care pediatric training center, the Clinical Practice Guideline Program has placed considerable emphasis on including residents, particularly interns, in the process of developing, implementing, and revising clinical practice guidelines. This approach encourages residents to use an evidence-based approach to practice. In addition, because interns play a critical role in care, engaging them in the clinical practice guideline process facilitates guideline implementation.

In response to an initially variable level of resident involvement, the chief medical resident and the director of the Clinical Practice Guideline Program convened a committee. This group sought to integrate clinical practice guidelines into house officer education and to involve house officers in all phases of clinical practice guideline development, implementation, and evaluation. The committee first surveyed medical interns to determine their level of involvement and general attitudes about guidelines. Survey results indicated that 89 percent of the interns agreed that clinical practice guidelines were designed to improve quality and 70 percent agreed that clinical practice guidelines at Children's Hospital, Boston, were designed to decrease costs.[8] Of the interns who were involved in clinical practice guideline development and implementation, all rated their clinical practice guideline involvement experience favorably. Although 74 percent of the interns had a favorable opinion of guidelines at Children's Hospital, Boston, some respondents expressed concerns about whether guidelines represented expert opinion, and, about how guidelines could affect physician autonomy. Although 100 percent of the clinical practice guidelines had involved interns, this involvement represented only 19 percent of the interns. Using these data and the recommendations from more experienced residents, the following interventions were implemented to improve resident participation:

1. Intern orientation is changed to include a brief introduction to clinical practice guidelines.
2. New interns are recruited to participate in ongoing clinical practice guideline activity starting the month after their internship begins.
3. Interns review the literature for their clinical practice guideline topic while serving on existing clinical practice guideline clinical working groups for the duration of their training. This arrangement allows the house officer to become expert in a particular topic while keeping the clinical working group up-to-date on that topic.
4. Clinical practice guidelines are being integrated into the core curriculum teaching sessions for residents. The chief medical resident oversees this aspect of integration.

At Children's Hospital, Boston, the chief medical residents are pivotal for the deployment of information on clinical practice guidelines. They coordinate communication to the house staff for the implementation of new clinical practice guidelines, integrate clinical practice guideline material into the intern orientation, and provide ongoing representation of residency training needs in relationship to clinical practice guideline activity. Most often, the residents in the clinical working group play a key role in communicating the information about a new clinical practice guideline, or a revision of an existing clinical practice guideline to their colleagues. Because Children's Hospital, Boston, is a teaching institution, the residents rotate every month between services and floors. During orientation to a given floor or unit, the nurse orienting the new residents reviews the clinical practice guidelines in use. The clinical working group resident will often attend intern rounds to present the clinical practice guideline.

Evidence- and Consensus-Based Recommendations Based on reviews of the adult literature, perhaps fewer than 20 percent of the clinical decisions are based on evidence.[9-13] In pediatrics the proportion of evidence-based practice is probably lower. While the Agency for Health Care Policy and Research and other national organizations often require a firm evidence base for their recommendations, using an evidence-based approach can be limiting when insufficient data exist; therefore, at Children's Hospital, Boston, a combination of literature review and consensus of expert opinion is used.[14] Some of our guidelines, which have been locally tailored from nationally developed guidelines, benefit from the comprehensive, critical literature reviews and the metanalyses completed for the national guideline. When a national guideline does not exist for a particular topic, every attempt is made to use existing evidence and consensus of expert opinion, because no single hospital has the resources to perform an evidence-based review with the same level of detail and methodological rigor as the Agency for Health Care Policy and Research or other national organizations. When acceptable evidence does not exist, review and discuss existing literature; gather information on pediatric practice patterns at other institutions through informal survey and networking; and use discussion, multivoting, and sometimes nominal group techniques to achieve consensus.[15-17]

Systems Thinking A system is an interdependent group of items, people, or processes with a common purpose.[18, 19] For each clinical practice guideline, the "system of care" for a specific diagnosis, condition, or technology is recognized before the scope of work for the clinical practice guideline is defined. When the continuum of care for the patient and family is acknowledged, it helps the participants to understand how the specific processes of care associated with the clinical practice guideline might complement or affect other aspects of care. For example, as the clinical working group identifies who is involved in the patient's care and how their involvement beyond the scope of the clinical practice guideline might affect its implementation, additional members may be identified and included in the clinical working group—for example, providers from the community or managed care organizations.

Multidisciplinary Approach We have found that the support and contribution of each clinical working group member is necessary to achieve successful implementation. Clinical working group members are selected to represent their perspective on the care of the patient being addressed by the clinical practice guideline.

There are two basic roles in the clinical working group. Core members of the clinical working group have expert knowledge of the clinical subject matter and experience or expert knowledge about the process of care associated with the use of the guideline. Consultant members are indirectly but significantly affected by the guideline and might have expertise needed by the clinical working group—for example, utilization review, case mix or finance expertise, administrative staff, etc. Consultants usually do not vote on clinical issues.

Clinician Ownership Ownership occurs when the clinical coleaders and clinical working group members assume responsibility for a clinical practice guideline and have a strong commitment to the clinical practice guideline's success. Usually this happens as a consequence of their participation in the clinical practice guideline process. If the clinical working group is locally tailoring a nationally established guideline, clinicians can achieve a sense of ownership for the clinical practice guideline and thereby improve the chances of successful implementation.[20-22] Most often this begins with clinician interest in and commitment to quality.

The presence of motivated leaders is perhaps the most important factor in assuring a clinical practice guideline's success. Most of our coleaders have been self-selected physicians and nurse managers or their designees. If the leaders demonstrate a sense of ownership through their motivation and leadership ability, they contribute to the sense of commitment on the part of the group. Clinical working members are encouraged to publish or present their work.

Identifying the Methods That Contribute to Successful Guidelines

Deploying a guideline does not always result in a measurable change in clinician behavior.[23-26] Following are some of the methods we believe contribute to successful guideline implementation in our setting. This is not intended to be a comprehensive description of our program, but rather a review of the clinical practice guideline process from the perspective of implementation. Key characteristics associated with implementation are described for each phase of the clinical practice guideline process—development, implementation, and evaluation.

Clinical Practice Guideline Development Following are the characteristics associated with implementation of the guideline development phase.

Clinical practice guideline topic selection: Of the selection criteria outlined in exhibit 8-1, clinician interest continues to be an important variable associated with implementation success. Clinician interest seems to be driven by the perceived need for improvement in clinical management.

The clinical practice guideline targets the care of the average, uncomplicated patient without major comorbidities and should have enough volume to allow for measurement. We usually recommend a volume of at least 50 or more discharges per year. Occasionally, high-cost, rare occurrence topics are considered—for example, use of extracorporeal membrane oxygenation. If the total number of patient days or patient visits averages around at least one patient per week, clinicians are more likely to remain aware of the clinical practice guideline.

Goal development: Having clearly stated goals enhances cooperation between clinical working group members, especially when there might be conflict of opinion or intrainstitutional competition—for example, among unit-based staff or specialties. G. J. Langley, K. M. Nolan, and T. W. Nolan identify cooperation in working toward a common goal as one of the key components associated with successful change.[27] To establish the goals and direction of the work, we use the following three questions required in the Langley model:

1. What are we trying to accomplish?
2. How will we know that a change is an improvement?
3. What changes can we make that will result in an improvement?[18]

Selection of the clinical working group: The size and the complexity of the clinical working group might affect clinical practice guideline development time and implementation. A larger group might be difficult to schedule, but a well-represented clinical working group might achieve a more successful implementation. The group size is usually a function of the complexity of the topic, the number of sites where the clinical practice guideline will be used, and the number of disciplines involved in care. The following examples demonstrate that group size and development time are not necessarily related.

In one case, a clinical working group developed a clinical practice guideline for the initial management of pleural effusion in the emergency department. Senior clinicians were concerned about the variation in management due to the number of physicians involved in care. Of particular concern was the timeliness of thoracentesis and drainage and variation in the diagnostic evaluation. The clinical working group consisted of 11 physicians, including residents, and 6 specialists and 1 nurse from the emergency department. An algorithm was developed and prepared for implementation in 5 meetings over 3 months.

In another case, the inpatient asthma clinical practice guideline dealt with key clinical decisions as well as the process of care for a diagnosis that involved multiple inpatient sites of care and required significant interdisciplinary collaboration. Although the clinical working group was a large, multidisciplinary group (28 members, 3 consultants), a comprehensive clinical practice guideline was developed in 12 meetings over 4 months and implemented on one unit. Within 18 months of implementation, the guideline had been evaluated, improved, and deployed throughout the medical units.

Definition of clinical practice guideline content: In developing the core content of the guideline, the process of care should be expressed as a flowchart, with the key clinical decisions for treatment and management noted. From this flowchart, the clinical working group will decide how to translate the recommendations for clinical decisions or processes into clinical care, and to identify the areas that will need to be targeted for implementation. In addition, through discussion of care process and clinical decisions, the clinical working group may identify others that need to be involved in the clinical practice guideline work to facilitate implementation.

Testing changes: While developing the clinical practice guideline, clinical working group members often identify unanticipated process problems that could create a barrier to the success of the clinical practice guideline. Usually a clinical working group member can begin gathering data to further define the problem or identify a possible solution. For example, the clinical working group developing the clinical practice guideline for ventricular–peritoneal shunt malfunction and infection realized early in the process of writing the clinical practice guideline that the neurosurgeons were using a variety of shunt drainage bags. With minimal research, an optimum, cost-effective drainage setup was selected and implemented even before the clinical practice guideline was completed.

Systems problems not unique to the clinical practice guideline: During the development or implementation of the clinical practice guideline, the clinical working group might identify process problems not unique to the clinical practice guideline, such as with the patient's experience of the care process—for example, waiting for an assessment, diagnostic test, or procedure; a system's problem; or general problems related to clinician behaviors—for example, documenting care, errors in procedures, etc.

For successful implementation, the clinical working group has to determine whether or not the problem can be resolved by the clinical working group and, if not, how to refer the problem for departmental or systemwide consideration. The Clinical Practice Guideline Program staff help the clinical working group to define the "boundaries" of clinical practice guideline work and identify resources for follow-up with a system's problems.

Translation of clinical practice guideline content into a clinical document: When creating clinical documents, the Clinical Practice Guideline Program adheres to two principles. First, clinicians are not asked to double-document. Second, clinical practice guideline documents should simplify work and clarify decisions. Currently, each clinical working group develops its own customized clinical practice guideline documents choosing one or more formats. These approaches might include the following:

- Decision aids

A flowchart or an algorithm works well for simple diagnoses when the goal of the clinical practice guideline is to reduce variation in clinical decision making. It provides a graphic stepwise description of the decisions specific to the diagnosis and management of a clinical problem.[28-31] We have implemented algorithms by setting up a process for the algorithm to be placed in the patient's record at the time the patient is identified as clinical practice guideline eligible or by making the algorithms accessible to the clinicians at the point of care. Index card summaries of the algorithms are being designed as pocket references for the physicians and nurses. Sometimes an algorithm is accompanied by or "nested in" a critical pathway. This method of combining decision aids with pathways has also been described by others.[32]

- Customized medical record documents

This method works well for high-volume diagnoses where multidisciplinary management of care is significant (for example, cystic fibrosis, bronchiolitis, and asthma). Approved medical record documents—such as physician order sheets, progress notes sheets, history and physical forms, and patient flowsheets—are customized by integrating the key elements of the clinical practice guideline into the medical record document. The greatest success has been with customized clinician order sheets. The effectiveness of preformatted medical record documents on clinician efficiency has been documented by others.[33]

- Annotations and references

Each key decision step of the clinical practice guideline is annotated with a brief discussion of the evidence. Acceptance of a clinical practice guideline by clinicians seems related to the perceived validity of the recommendations in the clinical practice guideline.[34, 35] For the clinical practice guideline to be successfully implemented, the users must understand the rationale for the recommendations.

Clinical Practice Guideline Implementation Following are the characteristics associated with the guideline implementation phase.

Planning for implementation: The implementation phase begins when the clinical practice guideline is deemed ready for clinical use. Planning for implementation might vary from developing a "to do" list based on careful discussion of all the decision nodes in the flowchart, to a more formal implementation plan as was developed for the inpatient asthma clinical practice guideline (exhibit 8-4). The clinical working group uses the flowchart of the care process to identify key steps that need to be included in the implementation plan. Each clinical working group member has a role in implementing the clinical practice guideline. Once the clinical practice guideline begins the implementation phase, the coleaders in their dual role as managers have the ability to solve problems when barriers are encountered.

Rapid cycle methods to test ideas prior to implementation: We have adapted a rapid cycle improvement method, described elsewhere by Langley and Nolan, for selected clinical practice guideline development and implementation. This method was used to implement a comprehensive, collaborative-model, short-stay program within the hospital.[36] The nursing director of this program subsequently decided to use the rapid cycle method to develop a clinical practice guideline for bronchiolitis, one of the most common diagnoses in the short-stay program.

The clinical practice guideline was developed in five meetings over the course of two months. The key idea with rapid cycle improvement is to identify an opportunity for improvement, rephrase the idea as a question—for example, "What will happen if . . . ?"—and then test it. Several ideas for improving the care process were tested on small samples of patients. The clinical documents, which included a flowchart of the patient care process and customized medical record documents (for example, physician order sheet, patient flowsheet, nursing and physician history and assessment form), were also tested on small samples. Clear measures for each goal were assessed and care was changed accordingly. The most notable improvements were decreasing the use of unnecessary oxygen saturation monitoring, basing clinical decisions on patient

EXHIBIT 8-4. Inpatient Asthma Clinical Practice Guidelines Implementation

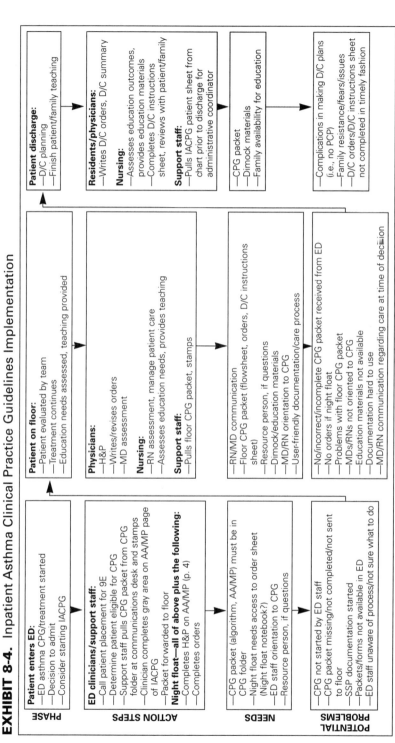

PHASE	**Patient enters ED:** —ED asthma CPG/treatment started —Decision to admit —Consider starting IACPG	**Patient on floor:** —Patient evaluated by team —Treatment continues —Education needs assessed, teaching provided	**Patient discharge:** —D/C planning —Finish patient/family teaching
ACTION STEPS	**ED clinicians/support staff:** —Call patient placement for 9E —Determine patient eligible for CPG —Support staff pulls CPG packet from CPG folder at communications desk and stamps —Clinician completes gray area on AA/MP page of IACPG —Packet forwarded to floor **Night float—all of above plus the following:** —Completes H&P on AA/MP (p. 4) —Completes orders	**Physicians:** —H&P —Writes/revises orders —MD assessment **Nursing:** —RN assessment, manage patient care —Assesses education needs, provides teaching **Support staff:** —Pulls floor CPG packet, stamps	**Residents/physicians:** —Writes D/C orders, D/C summary **Nursing:** —Assesses education outcomes, provides education materials —Completes D/C instructions sheet, reviews with patient/family **Support staff:** —Pulls IACPG patient sheet from chart prior to discharge for administrative coordinator
NEEDS	—CPG packet (algorithm, AA/MP) must be in CPG folder —Night float needs access to order sheet (Night float notebook?) —ED staff orientation to CPG —Resource person, if questions	—RN/MD communication —Floor CPG packet (flowsheet, orders, D/C instructions sheet) —Resource person, if questions —Dimock/education materials —MD/RN orientation to CPG —User-friendly documentation/care process	—CPG packet —Dimock materials —Family availability for education
POTENTIAL PROBLEMS	—CPG not started by ED staff —CPG packet missing/not completed/not sent to floor —SSP documentation started —Packets/forms not available in ED —ED staff unaware of process/not sure what to do	—No/incorrect/incomplete CPG packet received from ED —No orders if night float —Problems with floor CPG packet —MDs/RNs not oriented to CPG —Education materials not available —Documentation hard to use —MD/RN communication regarding care at time of decision	—Complications in making D/C plans (i.e., no PCP) —Family resistance/fears/issues —D/C orders/D/C instructions sheet not completed in timely fashion

assessment using a customized collaborative assessment tool, and minimizing the length of stay while improving patient satisfaction.[37]

This method of testing ideas as the clinical practice guideline is being developed is easiest to use with a straightforward, high-volume diagnosis implemented on one unit. However, this approach also has been useful in the development and implementation of more complex diagnoses. It requires skilled leadership, a clinical working group committed to working intensely over a specified amount of time, the ability to readily gather and analyze data to assess change, and a culture willing to innovate.

Education of clinicians and users: Educating the clinician and other users about a clinical practice guideline is one of the most important actions associated with successful implementation.[38] There are four principles that guide our approach to education.

First, a clinical practice guideline presentation should include the following:

- A discussion of the evidence and methods used to develop the clinical recommendations
- A review of the clinical practice guideline documents, noting who is responsible for their completion
- Clarification of how the clinical practice guideline document can be obtained
- Who can be called with questions or problems

Second, existing modes for communication, such as nursing reports, staff meetings, department meetings, medical and nursing rounds, resident teaching conferences, and existing committees, should be used to deploy a new clinical practice guideline. Children's Hospital, Boston's, nursing department has developed a deployment strategy for communicating new clinical information through the nursing education committee. This committee is successfully being used to keep nurses informed about new clinical practice guidelines. The chief resident's newsletter, a regular e-mail publication to residents about clinical issues, is used to deploy general clinical practice guideline information to residents.

Third, each clinical practice guideline is considered a work in progress and feedback on clinical content or format is requested from users by the clinical practice guideline coleaders, the clinical working group, and the Clinical Practice Guideline Program staff. We are currently working on accessible, user-friendly feedback methods.

Fourth, unless otherwise specified, each clinical practice guideline is considered a guideline that should inform practice, not a protocol that dictates practice. A standard paragraph emphasizing the guideline attribute and the need for clinicians to use their judgment based on the individual needs of the patient is included in every clinical practice guideline document.

Clinical Practice Guideline Evaluation The success of implementation is determined by evaluation. The clinical practice guideline evaluation should answer the following questions:

- Is the clinical practice guideline working as planned?
- Is there compliance with recommended practice?
- How has the clinical practice guideline affected outcomes?

These general questions are further refined with specific questions and measures and practically described in two phases: implementation appraisal and ongoing evaluation.

Implementation appraisal phase: The goal of the first few cycles of implementing the clinical practice guideline is to answer these questions: "Is the clinical practice guideline workable? Are the documents easy to use? Are there problems in the process, as defined by the clinical practice guideline, that need to be clarified or changed?"

Data are principally gathered through meeting with front-line users—that is, staff nurses, residents, and others—and through chart review by the clinical working group members of the first 10 or so patients. The former provides immediate feedback on all aspects of using the clinical practice guideline, and the latter allows assessment of compliance with key clinical practice recommendations.

Ongoing evaluation phase: These subsequent cycles of evaluation are intended to measure the effects of the clinical content on patient care process and clinical outcomes over time. Measures are determined based on the clinical practice guideline goals and are usually assessed in the implementation phase of the evaluation. Measures might include process of care variables, such as time from admission to first treatment, or success of communication with the primary care provider, and outcome variables including patient clinical outcomes, patient satisfaction, and resource consumption.

With each cycle of measurement, the clinical working group assesses the usefulness of each measure as an indicator of change—that is, "Did we make an improvement?" Reviewing of the clinical practice guideline goals and measures is done on a schedule specific to each clinical practice guideline. The clinical practice guideline should become a continuous learning process.

The timing and sample sizes for measurement vary for each clinical practice guideline and both of these factors can affect the momentum of implementation. For small-volume clinical practice guidelines (less than 100 per year), data are usually abstracted for key measures from the patient record for all patients. For larger clinical practice guidelines, a sampling method is used. If after reviewing the data the clinical working group decides to rapidly test a process revision, the clinical working group can collect data on all patients for a period of time to evaluate the change.

Data quality: Almost all hospital-based information systems have been established for billing and accounting purposes. Despite their accessibility, hospital data have a limited use in assessing clinical practice guideline effectiveness. If clinical practice guideline goals include reducing length of stay or variation in practices reliably captured by charge data, then the data are helpful.

However, many of the clinical and process improvement goals cannot be measured with case mix data. Often, clinical or process data need to be gathered through chart review or at the bedside. Utilization review staff resources can do concurrent chart review with clinical working group-designed audit tools. Occasionally, clinical working-group members have done retrospective chart review, particularly when data are needed on baseline or pre-clinical practice guideline patients or when data are needed on existing practices to inform clinical practice guideline development.

Research versus measurement for improvement: Early in the process of developing the clinical practice guideline, an attempt is made to distinguish those aspects of the clinical practice guideline that would constitute research and require an institutional review board approval process from those that are quality improvement activities and thus would not. The definition of research written by our institutional review board is used at times to help make the distinction. Also, our extensive experience with consumer surveys and quality improvement measurement helps to determine the status of a clinical practice guideline evaluation measure. If these issues are not clarified early in the process, it might not be possible to successfully implement the clinical practice guideline.

Assumptions about compliance: A key outcome measure of successful implementation is compliance. Compliance with a clinical practice guideline is encouraged but not mandated. The educational capacity and the quality benefits associated with improved care are emphasized to engage clinicians. Financial or disciplinary advantages have not been found to be associated with the use of enforced compliance methods and therefore were not used.[39] Evidence in the nuclear industry suggests that catastrophic consequences might result when the enforced use of standardized approaches exists in situations where the inputs are variable.[40] A level of necessary variation in clinical practice is anticipated and clinicians are advised to document all variances from a clinical practice guideline that has a rationale in the patient's record.

Mapping Areas for Future Growth

The process has identified three areas for future growth:

1. Automation

It is anticipated that implementation of guidelines will be greatly improved with an automated medical record and order entry. Our current information system includes a variety of distinct automated systems, and a basic order entry system is being piloted. However, to be successful, guideline automation needs to proceed cautiously in order not to arouse unrealistic expectations.[41]

2. Patient functional outcomes and patient/family satisfaction

Information from patients and/or families is obtained through survey or focus groups as appropriate for chronic diagnoses—for example, cystic fibrosis, asthma, and diabetes. For inpatient asthma, two outcomes survey samples are done per year. The data have been useful for improving patient teaching and discharge planning.

Our goal is to develop the resources for getting functional outcome data on clinical practice guideline patients. Although Children's Hospital, Boston, currently has both an inpatient and an outpatient consumer survey, the consumer survey data cannot be linked with clinical practice guideline patient populations because of the confidentiality barriers used to protect patient responses. Condition-specific consumer satisfaction and functional outcome data have been gathered for inpatient asthma and our goal is to expand this activity to other appropriate clinical practice guidelines.

3. Evaluation

We are improving our efficiency in developing clinical practice guideline measures and in collecting and analyzing data. Through repeated cycles of measurement, the most reliable and valid measures for each goal are retained and refined for the next cycle.

Summary

In the past four years, we have witnessed a major shift in attitudes about clinical practice guidelines at Children's Hospital, Boston. In the beginning, they were perceived as administratively imposed methods for reducing costs. Now clinical practice guidelines are seen as an opportunity to improve quality and decrease utilization. Clinical Practice Guideline Program staff continually have requests for new clinical practice guideline development. We believe this success can be attributed to the following aspects of our approach:

- Core programmatic support for clinical practice guideline work
- Involvement of residents in all aspects of clinical practice guideline activity
- A mixed evidence- and consensus-based approach
- Systems thinking
- Multidisciplinary approach
- Clinician ownership
- Focus on implementation throughout clinical practice guideline process

Two years into the program, the administrative structure for supervision of the Clinical Practice Guideline Program had outlived its usefulness. The Clinical Practice Guideline Steering Committee had accomplished its mission. The program was viewed as successful in its ability to support the development and implementation of clinical practice guidelines. The Clinical Practice Guideline Steering Committee was congratulated with cake and dissolved.

In addition, the Clinical Practice Guideline Steering Committee cochairs and Clinical Practice Guideline Program director recognized that the program needed to be integrated into operations. In the beginning, clinical practice guideline topics were reviewed and approved by the Clinical Practice Guideline Steering Committee. Now, department chairs and nursing directors are responsible for quality improvement activities for their department, including clinical practice guidelines. They are held accountable for their work to a hospitalwide, multidisciplinary committee responsible for quality. This model ensures that clinical practice guideline work is integrated into daily operations. However, the quality committee can directly delegate topics for clinical practice guideline development that are not "owned" by one department, yet are used throughout the hospital—for example, the use of expensive technologies, such as intravenous immunoglobulin. The Clinical Practice Guideline Program staff serve in a consultant role to department chairs and directors.

Clinical practice guidelines continue to evolve as a method to improve quality and manage costs. We believe our success has resulted from a variety of factors. We did not discuss, but highly recommend, the use of food to recognize the value of clinician time at meetings, being flexible at all times, and never losing one's sense of humor. Most important have been acknowledging a teaching hospital environment, involving pediatric residents, providing program support, using evidence- and consensus-based methods, and using a multidisciplinary approach.

References and Notes

1. Marilyn J. Field and Kathleen N. Lohr, eds., *Guidelines for Clinical Practice: From Development to Use* (Washington, DC: National Academy Press, 1992).

2. Richard J. Coffey, et al., "An Introduction to Critical Paths," *Quality Management in Health Care* 1, no. 1 (1992): 45-54.

3. D. S. Pare and M. D. Freed,"Clinical Practice Guidelines for Quality Patient-Outcome," in *The Nursing Clinics of North America Pediatric Collaborative Practice: A Cardiovascular Program,* Patricia A. Hickey, ed. (Philadelphia: Saunders, 1995), 30, no. 2, pp. 183-96.

4. P. Spevak, P. Moynihan, et al., "Clinical Practice Guidelines Can Reduce the Cost of Pediatric Cardiac Care [abstract]," in *Supplement to Circulation: Abstracts from the 66th Scientific Sessions of the American Heart Association,* Georgia, 1993, pp. I-532.

5. E. S. Rome, S. A. Moszczenski, et al., "A Clinical Pathway for Pelvic Inflammatory Disease for Use on an Inpatient Service," *Clinical Performance and Quality Health Care* 3, no. 4 (1995): 185-96.

6. The Harvard Community Health Plan has since merged with Pilgrim Health Care to become Harvard Pilgrim Health Care.

7. M. J. Field and K. N. Lohr, eds., *Guidelines for Clinical Practice: From Development to Use* (Washington, DC: National Academy Press, 1992).

8. R. G. Grossman, G. Priebe, J. Finkelstein, and D. Goldmann, "Integrating Clinical Practice Guidelines and Resident Training," Results, Eighth Annual National Forum on Quality Improvement in Health Care (New Orleans: Institute for Healthcare Improvement, 1996).

9. J. W. Williamson, P. G. Goldschmidt, and I. A. Jillson, "Medical Practice Information Demonstration Project: Final Report," Office of the Asst. Secretary of Health, DHEW, Contract #282-77-0068GS (Baltimore, MD: Policy Research, Inc., 1979).

10. J. P. Bunker, "Is Efficacy the Gold Standard for Quality Assessment?" *Inquiry* 25, no. 1 (1988): 51-8.

11. Institute of Medicine, *Assessing Medical Technologies* (Washington, DC: National Academy Press, 1985).

12. J. H. Ferguson, Foreword. *Research on the Delivery of Medical Care Using Hospital Firms,* Proceedings of a Workshop. April 30 and May 1, 1990, Bethesda, MD; *Med. Care* 29 (Suppl.) (1991): JS1-2.

13. M. Dubinsky and J. H. Ferguson, "Analysis of the National Institutes of Health Medicare Coverage Assessment," *Int. J. Technol. Health Care* 6, no. 3 (1990): 480-8.

14. M. J. Field and K. N. Lohr, Eds., "Building a Compelling Case for Recommendations," in *Guidelines for Clinical Practice: From Development to Use* (Washington, DC: National Academy Press, 1992), p. 7.

15. A. L. Delbecq, A. H. Van de Ven, and D. H. Gustafson, *Group Techniques for Program Planning: A Guide to Nominal Group and Delphi Processes* (Middleton, WI: Green Briar Press, 1986).

16. J. Lomas, "Words without Action? The Production, Dissemination, and Impact of Consensus Recommendations," *Ann. Rev. Publ. Health* 12 (1991): 41-65.

17. A. Fink, J. Kosecoff, M. R. Chassin, and R. H. Brook, "Consensus Methods: Characteristics and Guidelines for Use," *Am. J. Public Health* 74 (1984): 979-83.

18. G. J. Langley, K. M. Nolan, et al., *The Improvement Guide: A Practical Approach to Enhancing Organizational Performance* (San Francisco: Jossey-Bass, 1996), p. 7.

19. P. M. Senge, *The Fifth Discipline: The Art and Practice of the Learning Organization* (New York: Doubleday, 1990).

20. P. Bush, D. L. Rabin, and K. K. Spector, "Evaluation of a Drug Therapy Protocol in a Health Maintenance Organization," *Med. Care* 27 (1979): 566-77.

21. P. J. Greco and J. M. Eisenberg, "Changing Physicians Practices," *N. Engl. J. Med.* 329 (1993): 1271-3.

22. S. H. Woolf, "Practice Guidelines: A New Reality in Medicine," *Arch. Intern. Med.* 153 (1993): 2646-55.

23. W. M. Tierney, J. M. Overhage, C. J. McDonald, "Computerizing Guidelines: Factors for Success," Proceedings of the American Medical Informatics Association, 1996, Washington, DC.

24. M. N. Hill, D. M. Levine, and P. K. Whelton, "Awareness, Use and Impact of the 1984 Joint National Committee Consensus Report on High Blood Pressure," *Am. J. Pub. Health* 788 (1988): 1190-4.

25. J. Lomas, et al., "Do Practice Guidelines Guide Practice? The Effect of a Consensus Statement on the Practice of Physicians," *N. Engl. J. Med.* 321 (1989): 1306-11.

26. S. J. Cohen, M. Weinstein, S. L. Hui, W. M. Tierney, and C. J. McDonald, "The Impact of Reading on Physicians Nonadherence to Recommended Standards of Medical Care," *Soc. Sci. Med.* 21 (1985): 909-14.

27. G. J. Langley, K. M. Nolan, and T. W. Nolan, "The Foundation of Improvement," *Quality Progress* (June 1994): 81-6.

28. D. C. Hadorn, K. McCormick, and A. Diokno, "An Annotated Algorithm Approach to Clinical Guideline Development," *JAMA* 267, no. 24 (1992): 3311-4.

29. C. Z. Margolis, "Uses of Clinical Algorithms," *JAMA* 249, no. 5 (1983): 627-32.

30. L. K. Gottlieb, C. Z. Margolis, and S. C. Schoenbaum, "Clinical Practice Guidelines at a Health Maintenance Organization: Development and Implementation in a Quality Improvement Model," *QRB* 16 (1990): 80-6.

31. L. K. Gottlieb, H. N. Sokol, K. O. Murray, and S. C. Schoenbaum, "Algorithm-Based Clinical Quality Improvement: Clinical Guidelines and Continuous Quality Improvement," *Health Maintenance Organization Practice* 6, no. 1 (1992): 5-12.

32. J. Schriefer, "The Synergy of Pathways and Algorithms: Two Tools Work Better Than One," *J. Quality Improvement* 20, no. 9 (1994): 485-99.

33. T. Humphreys, F. S. Sofer, S. Jacobson, et al., "Preformatted Charts Improve Documentation in the Emergency Department," *Ann. Emergency Med.* 21 (1992): 534-40.

34. S. H. Woolf, "Practice Guidelines, a New Reality in Medicine. II. Methods of Developing Guidelines," *Arch. Intern. Med.* 152 (1992): 946-52.

35. J. B. Brown, D. Shye, and B. McFarland, "The Paradox of Guideline Implementation: How AHCPR's Depression Guideline Was Adapted at Kaiser Permanente Northwest Region," *J. Quality Improvement* 21, no. 1 (1995): 5-21.

36. P. A. Rutherford, "Rapid Cycle Changes in Clinical Care," Institute for Healthcare Improvement, National Forum on Quality Improvement in Health Care Results, 1996, p. 33; Langley, Nolan et al., *The Improvement Guide.*

37. P. Rutherford, "Rapid Cycle Changes in Clinical Practice Guideline Development," Proceedings of MassPRO's 2nd Annual Health Care Quality Summit, Nov. 13, 1996, Burlington, MA.

38. J. B. Rischer and S. B. Childress, "Cancer Pain Management: Pilot Implementation of the AHCPR Guideline in Utah," *J. Quality Improvement* 22, no. 10 (1996): 683-99.

39. S. H. Woolf, "Practice Guidelines: A New Reality in Medicine," *Arch. Intern. Med.* 153 (1993): 2646-55.

40. C. Perrow, *Normal Accidents* (New York: Basic Books, 1984).

41. Tierney et al., "Computerizing Guidelines."

SUMMARY COMMENTS FOR THE CASE STUDIES

Although the Kaiser Permanente, Georgia, story is about a health maintenance organization guidelines program and the Children's Hospital, Boston, story is about a teaching hospital program, the similarities between these stories are certainly much stronger than the differences. These similarities can be summarized as follows:

- Motivation: The financial performance was suboptimal. At Kaiser Permanente, Georgia, there were too many referrals and too many lab tests; at Children's Hospital, Boston, the length of stay was too long and there were too many lab tests; in both clinical settings, the aim was to improve quality by decreasing unnecessary variation in clinical practice across clinicians.
- Quality improvement context: This was the conceptual basis for developing and subsequently implementing clinical practice guidelines.
- Create a central organizational unit: The organizational structure of the program was similar in that both settings established a

central support unit and appointed a clinician-administrator leadership team.
- Leadership by a clinician-administrator team: (see above)
- Guideline development:
  —Use both consensus-based and evidence-based techniques
  —Use a multidisciplinary team to develop guidelines.
  —Insure updating.
  —Monitor provider satisfaction with guidelines.
- Evaluation:
  —Start evaluation planning when finishing guidelines.
  —Monitor both process and outcome.
- Develop a dissemination and learning plan: As indicated in the guidelines bi-cycle, dissemination and learning were planned, not left to chance.
- Implementation:
  —Start planning implementation when finishing guideline development.
  —Use the cheapest implementation strategy
  —Involve patients in determining implementation problems and solutions.
  —Use automated reminders.

Instructive differences between these two approaches to implementation of a guidelines program are as follows: At Kaiser Permanente, Georgia, there was a strong emphasis on referral management In the guidelines. At Children's Hospital, Boston, residents were involved in every step of guideline development, dissemination, implementation, and using a rapid cycle method of piloting and then testing implementation steps. Also, contracting with a major health maintenance organization was a strong motivating factor in getting the program started.

The Transient Ischemic Attack Files: An Implementation Case Study

Nancy Sokol, MD

This exercise is designed to walk you through the principal elements of guideline implementation that you have learned thus far. The exercise presents a hypothetical case study in which a guideline is to be implemented to manage patients with transient ischemic attack. It is divided into steps of guideline planning, implementation, and monitoring. Questions are presented to simulate those that might arise when you are working in similar situations in the clinical setting. A discussion of answers will follow in this appendix.

After following this exercise, you should have an understanding of the following skills:

- Evaluating data to determine where to focus a clinical improvement effort
- Recognizing the role of a process flowchart in identifying outcomes and need for clinical guidelines
- Learning strategies to identify barriers to guideline adoption and to direct implementation efforts to overcome those barriers
- Understanding the relationship between guidelines and clinical pathways
- Targeting measures based on a clinical algorithm and clinical pathway
- Interpreting samples of outcomes data

THE EXERCISE

Defining the Project

You are chairperson of the neurology department in a 200-bed community hospital. Facing potential extinction in the highly competitive world of hospitals, and somewhat at odds with several outspoken members of the medical staff, your hospital director has recently negotiated to participate in a Medicare risk contract, Healthy Maturity. The hospital will receive capitated funds for enrolled seniors in the cachement area and now stands to benefit from reducing hospital admissions, lengths of stay, and costs for patients in this program. Because of greatly reduced premiums, a large senior enrollment is anticipated. Almost all of the hospital physicians will participate. Healthy Maturity, in agreement with Medicare, will be monitoring patient satisfaction and health outcomes. You, along with other hospital chairs, have been charged with the responsibility of developing a program within your department which will impact the costs of disease management for the Medicare population.

- Question 1: Who are the customers for this project? Who are the suppliers? Why are these factors critical?

Your customer (hospital administrator) makes it clear that the primary objectives for your project should be to decrease hospitalization rates and length of stay. Your other customers (Healthy Maturity and enrolled patients) want to ensure that quality of care is maintained while costs are addressed.

- Question 2: What data would you wish to review in order to select a neurologic condition on which to focus?

Stroke and transient ischemic attack are the two most common admitting diagnoses in neurology for this older population. Stroke occurs when there has been infarction of brain tissue, due to thrombosis, embolism, or intracerebral bleeding. Patients who have suffered recent strokes require hospitalization for monitoring and interventions aimed at limiting the extent of neurologic deficit.

The transient ischemic attack is a condition of temporary lack of blood supply to the brain. This results in a neurologic deficit (such as loss of speech, inability to move an extremity) which resolves completely, usually in a few minutes and by definition always in less than 24 hours. The lack of blood supply is due either to critical narrowing of the arteries supplying the brain or to an embolus which has dislodged from within the heart and migrated into the brain. Unlike a stroke, the affected area of the brain recovers completely, either because of collateral blood supply or because the embolus breaks up. The main significance of a transient ischemic attack is that it is a warning that further cardio-vascular events (stroke or heart attacks) might occur, and treatment for transient ischemic attack is really treatment to prevent such future events. The same patient population, more or less, is at risk for both stroke and transient ischemic attack. The data shown in table A-1 and figures A-1 through A-3 were part of the set generated by your hospital information system.

TABLE A-1. Admitting Diagnoses to Neurology Service, Patients over 65 Years of Age

Diagnosis	No. Patients	Average Length of Stay	Neurologist	No. Patients	Average Length of Stay
Stroke	160	5.1 d	A	23	5.3
			B	27	5.1
			C	44	4.9
			D	25	5.2
			E	16	4.9
			F	25	5.0
TIA	103	4.3 d	A	20	4.2
			B	7	3.1
			C	27	6.1
			D	25	2.8
			E	17	4.9
			F	7	2.6

FIGURE A-1. Admissions

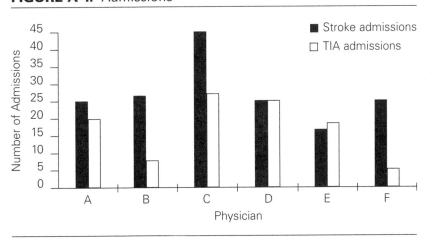

FIGURE A-2. Length of Stay for Stroke (N = 160)

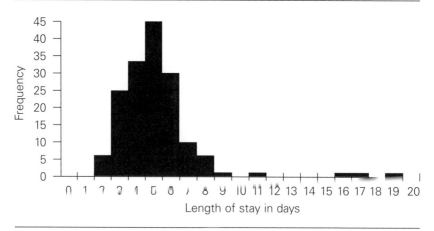

Length of stay in days

FIGURE A-3. Length of Stay for Transient Ischemic Attack (N = 103)

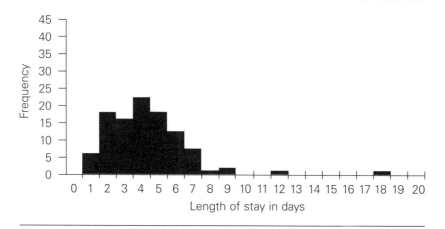

Length of stay in days

- Question 3: What might you hypothesize about the practices or practice styles of neurologists B, C, D, and F? What can you say about the length of stay for stroke compared to that for transient ischemic attack?

Considering that not all patients with transient ischemic attack are admitted to the hospital, you realize that the data you have reviewed so far only reflect hospitalized patients.

- Question 4: How can you identify those transient ischemic attack patients managed by your staff neurologists who were not hospitalized? Why is this important?

Initiating a Guideline

Based on your review of the data, you decided to organize a project aimed at management of patients with transient ischemic attack (see figure A-4). You notified your staff that their next monthly meeting would be devoted to a discussion of appropriate management of patients with transient ischemic attack. A heated debate quickly ensued. Dr. Articule was very disturbed that a patient of his had been seen in the emergency room by another neurologist, was discharged on aspirin without being hospitalized, and had a complete stroke the following day. "He should never have been sent home without anticoagulation!" he exclaimed. Dr. Blate had just been notified that a patient of his, who had been anticoagulated for a transient ischemic attack several months earlier, had suffered a brain hemorrhage and died. "He should never have been on anticoagulants—aspirin is safer and more effective!" he, in turn, exclaimed.

It became clear that it would take more than a one-hour meeting to bring your staff to agreement on strategies for managing transient ischemic attack. While there was marked disagreement on factors to be weighed in making specific clinical decisions, your staff did agree that the following "high-level process flow" outlined the general management strategy for patients presenting with possible transient ischemic attack.

The following points will be helpful for those readers who have not used process flowcharts:

- A process flowchart is a graphical representation of the sequence of steps in a process. In the health care setting, it can define patient flow, information flow, and material flow.

FIGURE A-4. Management of Transient Ischemic Attack

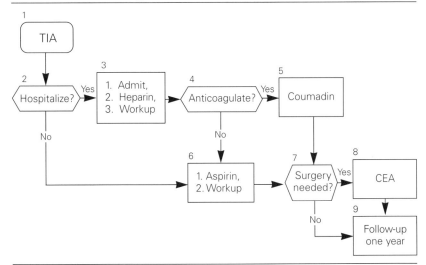

- A high-level process flow has fewer than 10 to 12 boxes and can be greatly expanded. Contained with the high-level flow are multiple detailed flowcharts and often, in the health care setting, several clinical algorithms.
- Symbols used in process flow charts are the same as those for clinical algorithms, with a few additional symbols, including the following:

    — ▢ Wait: point of delay in process

    — ☁ Cloud: process not well defined (often a cloud denotes an area where a clinical guideline might be helpful)

- Question 1: Is the process diagrammed in figure A-4 a clinical guideline? If not, why not? Where are the "wait points" and "cloud points" in this process?

This process flow, while not "guiding" care, is useful in two ways: it helps to highlight where the controversies are and where guidelines would be needed; and it helps to define starting and ending points for the process to guide measurement strategies.

- Question 2: How many potential points of clinical decision making are indicated by this process flow? How many pathways are there in this guideline?

- Question 3: Given this process flow scheme and what you've been told of the outcomes of patients with transient ischemic attack, what intermediate and final outcomes would you want to measure? Which patients should be studied for these outcomes?

The group of neurologists started to feel a bit better about the transient ischemic attack project when they realized there were some big picture components on which they could easily agree. They then decided to address the controversial issues regarding indications for hospitalization and anticoagulation. They felt that decisions about appropriateness for surgery would best be addressed by the vascular surgeons and neurosurgeons and you agreed to convene a second team to develop guidelines for carotid endarterectomy. However, Dr. Articule and Dr. Blate were not interested in working on the guidelines.

- Question 4: How might you engage their participation?

Developing the Guideline

In gathering data for your transient ischemic attack project, you discover that neurology is only one (although the most common) of seven services which admits transient ischemic attack patients (see figure A-5).

- Question 1: What impact will this have on developing a guideline at your staff meeting? What impact will this have on implementing a guideline?

Literature was reviewed, and the result was varying opinions on whether patients with transient ischemic attack should be anticoagulated. The group decided to review only the evidence from original, randomized trials on the outcomes of treatment with anticoagulation (Heparin followed by Coumadin) versus those of treatment with aspirin. There were only two such studies. Neither study showed an advantage to Coumadin, except in patients who had a cardiac source for embolus. This was a surprise to several of the physicians, whose assumption had always been that aspirin, while safer and not requiring the close monitoring that is required for Coumadin, was not as effective as Coumadin.

If routine anticoagulation requiring intravenous Heparin while awaiting therapeutic Coumadin levels was not needed, then hospitalization was indicated only for a subset of transient ischemic attack patients. The guidelines team used a consensus process to develop criteria for hospitalization and eventually issued a guideline with logic presented in the clinical algorithm shown in figure A-6.

FIGURE A-5. Transient Ischemic Attack by Discharge Service (N=151)

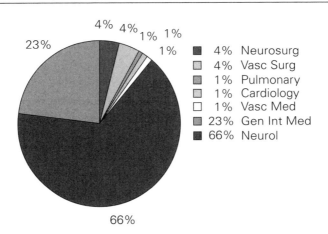

4%	Neurosurg
4%	Vasc Surg
1%	Pulmonary
1%	Cardiology
1%	Vasc Med
23%	Gen Int Med
66%	Neurol

FIGURE A-6. Management of Transient Ischemic Attacks

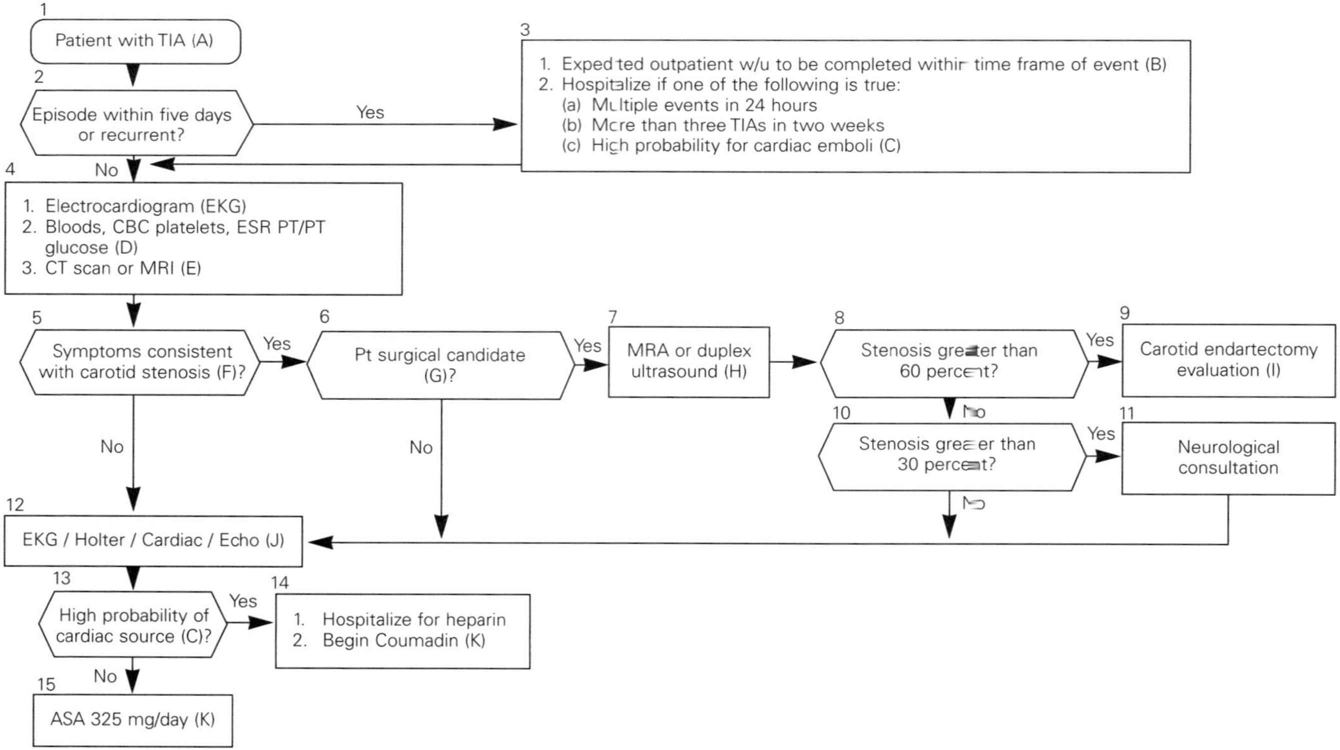
1
Patient with TIA (A)
2
Episode within five days or recurrent?
Yes
3
1. Expedited outpatient w/u to be completed within time frame of event (B)
2. Hospitalize if one of the following is true:
(a) Multiple events in 24 hours
(b) More than three TIAs in two weeks
(c) High probability for cardiac emboli (C)
4
No
1. Electrocardiogram (EKG)
2. Bloods, CBC platelets, ESR PT/PT glucose (D)
3. CT scan or MRI (E)
5
Symptoms consistent with carotid stenosis (F)?
Yes
6
Pt surgical candidate (G)?
Yes
7
MRA or duplex ultrasound (H)
8
Stenosis greater than 60 percent?
Yes
9
Carotid endartectomy evaluation (I)
No
10
Stenosis greater than 30 percent?
Yes
11
Neurological consultation
No
No
No
12
EKG / Holter / Cardiac / Echo (J)
13
High probability of cardiac source (C)?
Yes
14
1. Hospitalize for heparin
2. Begin Coumadin (K)
No
15
ASA 325 mg/day (K)

Implementing the Guideline

The first step was to perform an operational analysis. The guideline was reviewed and endorsed by the chairpersons of neurology, internal medicine, neurosurgery, vascular surgery, cardiology, and radiology.

- Question 1: Is this review sufficient to ensure that the recommendations will be able to be implemented with appropriate decision supports? If not, what further steps could be taken?

An operational analysis of the transient ischemic attack guideline led to recognition of the following: In order for the outpatient workup to be completed on the weekend in a suitable time frame, the lab that performs carotid studies needed to be staffed with on-call personnel.

Magnetic resonance imaging and magnetic resonance angiography availability in short time frames was not currently implementable, but arrangements were in place to purchase a new magnetic resonance machine for the hospital. Current contracts with outside vendors would need to be negotiated to improve urgent access.

Moreover, emergency room space was limited, and patients who previously would have been admitted into the hospital and removed from the emergency room quickly now would need to be housed for a least one to two hours for their workup. Because the hospital census was down, there were vacant beds elsewhere that could have been used for short-term "observation" status. Protocols would need to be developed in order to select appropriate patients for this status, and in order to staff and monitor these beds.

Key to guideline implementation is identifying the potential barriers to clinician adoption of the guideline recommendations and developing specific implementation strategies to overcome these barriers. There are several possible strategies to identify barriers, including the following:

- Brainstorming with a group of potential guideline users
- Identification of essential and controversial nodes, in either the guideline or the flowchart
- Failure mode effects analysis
- Force field analysis

We will practice the last two of these.

Failure mode effects analysis is a technique borrowed from industries designing critical pieces of hardware (such as airplanes) and is used for protection against design failures. Each process activity (each algorithm box) is evaluated for potential failure, and possible causes of failure are predicted. A rating is given to each cause, based on the likelihood of the failure occurring and the severity of its impact on the overall process. This gives rise to rank ordering of potential causes of failure and, therefore, prioritization of areas at which to aim implementation supports.

The failure mode effects analysis grid shown in table A-2 is completed for box 2 and box 3, part 1, of the guideline.

- Question 2: Consult the guideline and try your hand at completing part 2 of box 3.

With regard to force field analysis, Lomas categorizes five influences on clinical decision making: patient factors, personal factors, educational factors, administrative issues, and economic considerations. As shown in figure A-7, Handley and Stuart from Group Health Cooperative of Puget Sound suggest considering how each of these factors can drive or restrain adoption of guideline recommendations, and term this analysis creating a "force field diagram."

- Question 3: Try to list the force field factors for adoption of the transient ischemic attack guideline.

The preceding analyses led to recognition of the need to design decision supports. Following are major barriers of guideline adoption:

- Resistance of medical doctors
- Emergency room unavailable to house patient for immediate workup
- Diagnostic studies not available off hours
- Patient expectation for hospitalization

Decision supports can be categorized in the following manner:

- Educational
- Administrative
- Reminders and feedback
- Incentives

- Question 4: Think about possible decision support strategies, referring to the barriers identified by the failure mode effects analysis and force field diagram, considering multiple, and even fanciful, interventions.

Developing a Clinical Care Path

Within three months of implementation, the guideline had made a significant impact on the hospital admission rate. However, the length of stay for those patients being admitted remained unaffected. A clinical care pathway was developed.

TABLE A-2. Partially Completed Failure Mode Effects Analysis Table

Process Step	Potential Failure Mode	Possible Causes	Likelihood (L) (1–5)	Severity (S) (1–5)	Priority (L x S) (1–25)	Overall Effect
2. TIA (5d) or recurrent	Don't identify new TIA patient	Doctor not aware important	1	3	3	High recurrence TIA or stroke
		Patient denies	1		3	High recurrence TIA or stroke
	Don't identify recurrent TIA patient	Doctor not aware important	2	4	8	High recurrence TIA or stroke
		Patient denies	1		4	High recurrence TIA or stroke
3.1 Expedited outpatient workup	Workup takes too long	Tests unavailable	4	3	12	High recurrence TIA or stroke
		Not ordered appropriately	2		6	High recurrence TIA or stroke
	Workup takes too long	Patient didn't keep appointment	1	3	3	High recurrence TIA or stroke

187

FIGURE A-7. Force Field Diagram

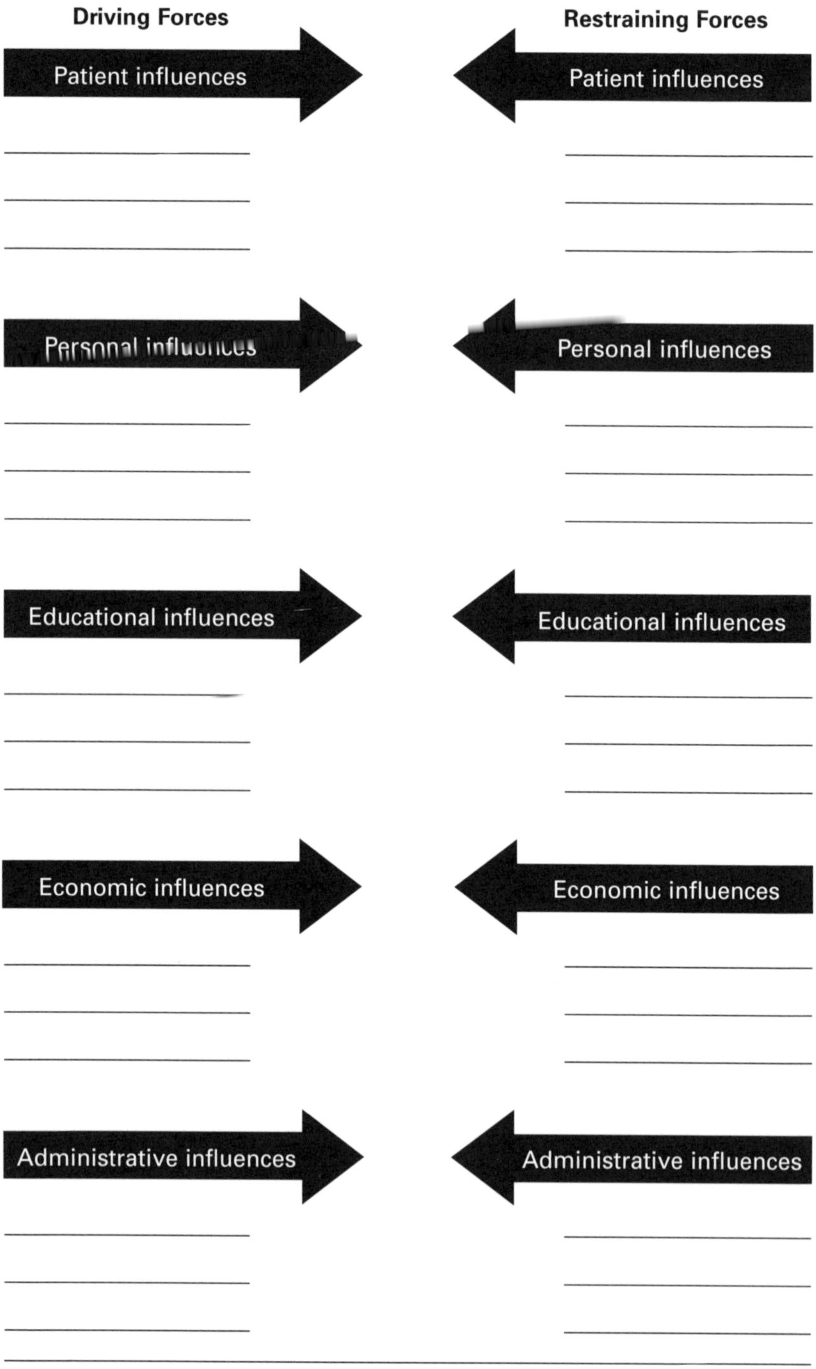

- Question 1: Who should participate on this team? Why is this team composition different from a guidelines team?

The team used a consensus process to develop the path shown in table A-3 for patients hospitalized for transient ischemic attack.

- Question 2: How does this path differ from the clinical algorithm? How is it the same? Is it always necessary to have a guideline before a clinical path? What are the essential elements in the clinical path that are not present in the process flow or guideline?

- Question 3: What procedures would you follow to implement this clinical pathway?

Interpreting Data, Revising the Pathway, Spin-off Projects

Data were collected one year after transient ischemic attack guideline implementation. A database was set up to identify all patients with transient ischemic attack managed by the hospital physicians, to include both ambulatory and in-hospital patients (patients were identified at the time of their computed tomography or magnetic resonance imaging). Since this database did not exist prior to the guideline, a pre–post comparison of clinical practice patterns and patient outcomes could not be accomplished. Data became available to examine the following:

- Hospitalization rates
- Length of stay
- Anticoagulation rates
- Diagnostic tests ordered
- Surgery rates
- Outcomes
  —Neurologic
  —Cardiac
  —Treatment complications
  —Mortality
- Hospital charges

In terms of hospitalization length of stay for transient ischemic attack patients in neurology, data were prepared to compare neurology practices before and after implementation of the guideline and clinical pathway (see figures A-8 through A-11).

- Question 1: What can you conclude about the impact of the implementation strategies on decisions to admit patients with transient ischemic attack, and their length of stay?

TABLE A-3. Clinical Pathway—Transient Ischemic Attack

	Day 1 ER Admit	Day 2	Day 3	Day 4	Day 5 Discharge by 10 a.m.	Outcomes (Variance code needed for delayed discharge)
Consultation	Neurology Medicine if needed	Social service, vascular surgery if needed				
Tests/Specimens	1. CT Head 2. Labs 3. EKG 4. MRA or NICS	1. TE Echo if needed 2. Holter if needed 3. Arteriogram if needed 4. PT/PTT if needed				
Treatments			Carotid endarterectomy if needed	Switch pathway		Patient will be on oral medication
Medications	Heparin if needed within 12 hours of admission	1. Coumadin decision Ordered as needed: a. Coumadin b. Heparin c. ASA d. Tictopidine	Order as needed: Coumadin Heparin	Order as needed: Coumadin Heparin	Order as needed: Coumadin Heparin	
Diet		Regular	Regular	Regular	Regular	
Elimination	Ad lib					
Activity						
Education		1. Begin teaching: a. Coumadin b. S&S of TIA	Reinforce	Reinforce	Reinforce	
Discharge planning		1. Evaluate need for home care services 2. Evaluate meds for discharge	1. Arrange for PT training 2. Formulate home care instruction sheet 3. Review with patient and significant others 4. Notify required agency			Patient will be discharged with necessary support services

FIGURE A-8. Comparison of Admissions, Before Implementation

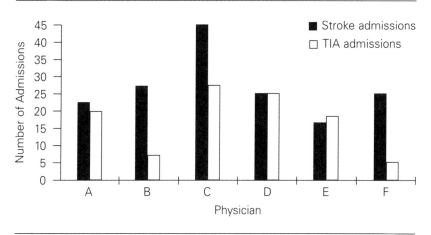

FIGURE A-9. Comparison of Admissions, After Implementation

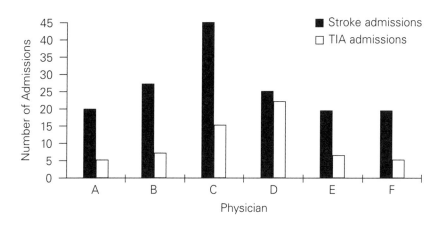

In terms of patient outcomes, data were collected on the clinical outcomes of patients with transient ischemic attack, followed up one year postevent. Tables A-4 and A-5 show the information that was obtained.

The data suggest that patients admitted to the hospital had significantly more adverse events than did patients who were not admitted.

- Question 2: What hypotheses might explain this? What additional data would you like to consider in order to interpret these findings?

FIGURE A-10. Length of Stay for Transient Ischemic Attack (N = 103), Before Implementation

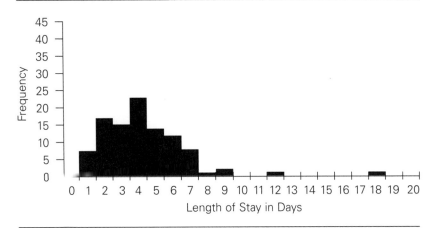

Length of Stay in Days

FIGURE A-11. Length of Stay for Transient Ischemic Attack (N = 86), After Implementation

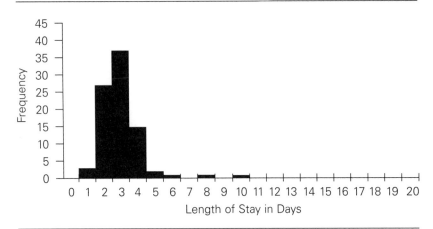

Length of Stay in Days

TABLE A-4. Number of Patients with and without Adverse Events

Admitted to Hospital?	Any adverse events?		
	No	Yes	Total
No	197	29	226
Yes	56	19	75
Total	253	48	301

Pearson chi-sqare (1) = 6.5659   Pr = 0.010
Fisher's exact test = 0.017
One-tail Fisher's exact test = 0.010

One concern raised was that patients who were hospitalized were more likely to be placed on long-term anticoagulation and that perhaps the increased morbidity of these patients was related to the anticoagulation. See the data in table A-6.

- Question 2: Do these data support the hypothesis that Coumadin use explains the increase in adverse events? Do the above data suggest that the guideline or clinical pathway needs to be revised?

TABLE A-5. Number of Patients, by Type of Complication

Type of Complication	Admitted to Hospital?		
	No	Yes	Total
None	197	56	253
Stroke alone	6	3	9
Stroke + TIA	0	1	1
Stroke + MIA	0	2	2
MIA alone	2	3	5
MI + TIA	0	1	1
TIA alone	21	5	26
TIA + Coum Comp	0	1	1
Coum Comp alone	0	2	2
Death	0	1	1
Total patients	226	75	301

TABLE A-6. Adverse Events from Coumadin Use

Coumadin on D/C?	Any adverse events?		
	No	Yes	Total
No	19	4	23
Yes	37	15	52
Total	56	19	75

Pearson chi-sqare (1) = 1.1062   Pr = 0.293
Fisher's exact test = 0.393
One-tail Fisher's exact test = 0.225

While the length of stay was reduced for hospitalized patients, there was still significant variation, suggesting further room for improvement. The measurement team looked at factors that might impact the length of stay, and found that the strongest correlation was with the day Coumadin was introduced and how long it took to achieve therapeutic anticoagulation on a stable Coumadin dose.

- Question 3: Given this finding, what further actions might be taken? Does this suggest that the guideline or clinical pathway needs to be revised?

Two spin-off projects were initiated, as systems improvement projects. A heparinization team developed a protocol to rapidly and safely achieve therapeutic heparin levels, based on a recently published article. An oral anticoagulation team developed a program within the hospital, run by a dedicated nurse, to track, monitor, and make dose adjustments by telephone for patients who were discharged on Coumadin. This was welcomed by the hospital physicians as a needed service providing relief for them from the hassles of adjusting the medication and fear of litigation (anticoagulation errors being a frequent issue in malpractice).

REVIEW

Referring to the guidelines bi-cycle shown in figure FM-1 at the beginning of the book, you can see that the transient ischemic attack project from beginning to end illustrates the following steps:

- Transient ischemic attack project identification
- Transient ischemic attack guideline development (part of the guideline development cycle)
- Barrier detection
- Decision support design
- Implementation plan development (implied, though not actually shown)
- Evaluation plan development (implied, though not actually shown)
- Pilot
- Implementation and evaluation

SUMMARY

A case is presented in which a hospital department is asked to focus on a clinical condition (transient ischemic attack) and develop a program that will result in decreasing hospital costs. Data are reviewed to select an appropriate clinical topic, and a team of clinicians is convened. A process flow scheme is drawn, which highlights outcomes of care to be measured.

Despite controversy, a transient ischemic attack guideline is developed, based on evidence from the literature and consensus, and it is examined for potential barriers to its implementation. Implementation strategies and decision supports are developed to foster compliance with the guideline, which is anticipated to decrease hospitalization rates.

Hospitalization rates indeed begin to drop, but length of stay remains unchanged. A second team is convened to address shortening hospital stays by developing and implementing a clinical care pathway. Implementation and measurement strategies based on the care pathway are proposed.

Finally, outcomes data are evaluated in order to help make sense of the impact of the guideline and pathway implementation. Revision of the pathway is recommended, and need for a process improvement project is identified. Two projects (oral anticoagulation team and hospitalization team) are implemented.

ANSWERS

Defining the Project

1. The customers are the hospital administrator, Healthy Maturity patients, and Healthy Maturity administration and medical director. The suppliers are you, your staff, and all hospital personnel involved in management of patients. Note the customer/supplier chain. Patients are customers supplied by Healthy Maturity, a customer of hospital administration, which is in turn a customer of the neurology department. Healthy Maturity is a supplier to patients (and to the Department of Health and Human Services!), the hospital administration is a supplier to Healthy Maturity, and the neurology department supplies to hospital administration (as do laboratory services to neurology!). Only patients seem not to be suppliers, while laboratory services seem not to be customers (or are they?).

It is important to recognize customers who do the following:

- Determine customer needs
- Determine outcome preferences
- Authorize resource delegation (staff time, supplies, data)
- Suppliers need to be involved in designing and maintaining a process of care that will meet customer needs.

2. You might want to consider the following data (the list is not all-inclusive):

- Rank order or neuro diagnosis-related groups for patients more than 65 years of age by the following measures:
  —Admitting diagnosis
  —Length of stay
  —Costs
- Variation in length of stay
- Variation in costs
- Variation in number or cost of diagnostic studies ordered
- Variation in hospital admission rates by neurologist

It is important to recognize that unexplained variation is important to identify, since it indicates that there is the potential opportunity to identify a best practice and modify existing practice. Where there is no variation, it is possible that current practice is already optimal, even for diagnoses where there are high costs (although it is also possible that clinicians are uniformly practicing suboptimally!).

3. It is easier to interpret the data from figures A-1 and A-2. Neurologist B has a practice that is average for stroke admissions, but hospitalizes relatively few patients with transient ischemic attack. Neurologist C hospitalizes an average number of patients with transient ischemic attack, but probably has a larger patient base, which suggests he selects patients for transient ischemic attack admissions. Neurologist D hospitalizes as many transient ischemic attack patients as she does stroke patients—does she hospitalize all her transient ischemic attack patients? Neurologist E has a practice pattern like that of D, though fewer patients; Neurologist F has a practice pattern like that of B.

The histogram for length of stay shows a normal distribution for stroke, with a few outliers. There is more of a plateau shape for transient ischemic attack, which suggests either that there is no process or that there are multiple processes impacting length of stay. These data suggest that there is considerable variability both in decisions to admit patients with transient ischemic attack and in hospital management once patients are admitted.

4. You could see if your neurologists maintain their own data bases on patients they see. In addition, you could try to track patients through your laboratory services, assuming there is one lab test, at one site, that patients would get, whether they are hospitalized or not (for example, computed tomography scan).

This is important because it is essential to look at the universe of patients with transient ischemic attack, not just patients hospitalized with the condition, in order to determine the hospitalization rates, outcomes, costs of care, and variation in care for the entire population.

FIGURE A-12. Management of Transient Ischemic Attack

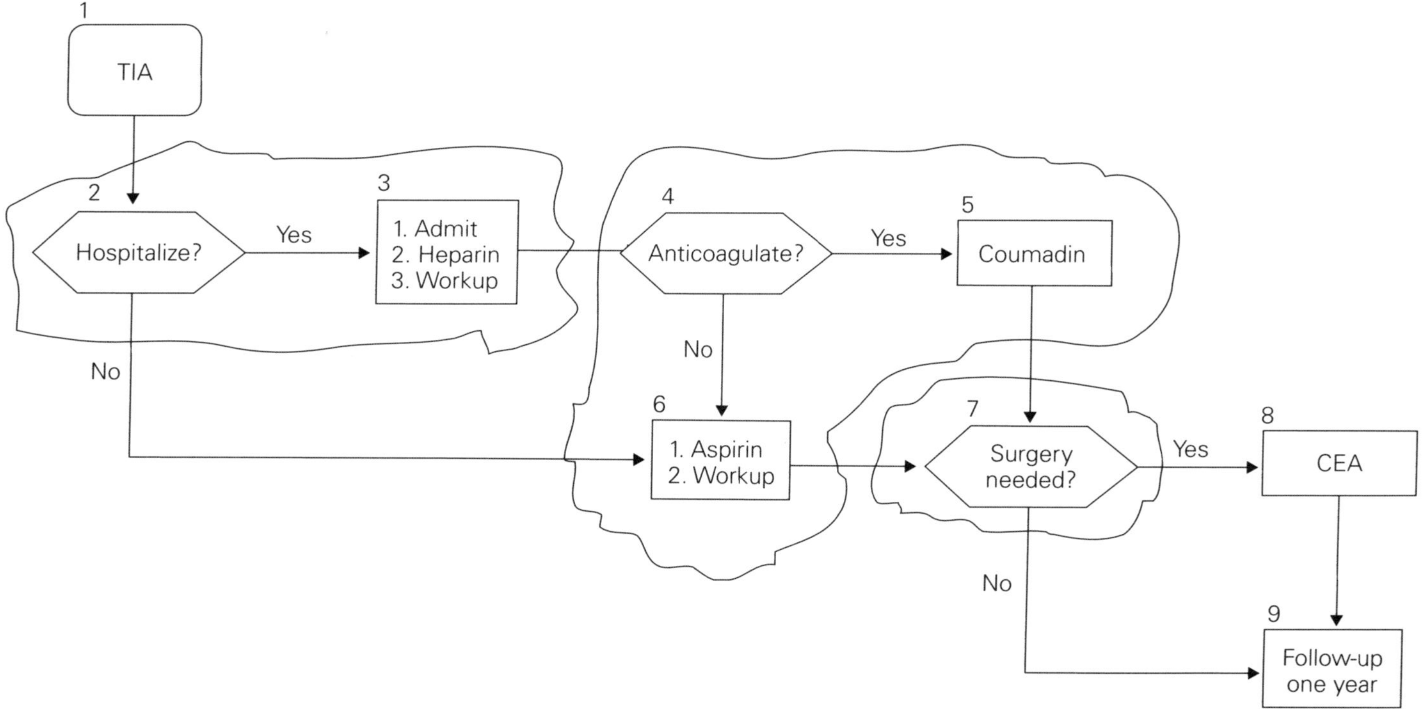

Initiating a Guideline

1. "Wait points" and "cloud points" are noted on the flowchart in figure A-12. This would not work as a clinical guideline, as it doesn't give any information about how to make the clinical decisions: when to hospitalize, when to anticoagulate, who should have surgery, what workup to perform. Given to a group of neurologists, it would not result in reproducible patient evaluations or management strategies.

2. As figure A-12 shows, there are three points of clinical decision making (that is, "cloud" states) for which a clinical guideline might be helpful:

- Whether to hospitalize
- Whether to anticoagulate
- Whether to refer for surgery

There are six possible pathways for this flowchart:

- 1,2,3,4,5,7,8,9
- 1,2,3,4,5,7,9
- 1,2,3,4,6,7,8,9
- 1,2,3,4,6,7,9
- 1,2,6,7,8,9
- 1,2,6,7,9

3. The process flowchart in figure A-12 helps to identify important intermediate outcomes, as follows:

- Percentage of patients with transient ischemic attack who were hospitalized
- Percentage of patients with transient ischemic attack who were anticoagulated
- Percentage of patients with transient ischemic attack who had surgery

At the one-year follow-up, you would want to determine the clinical status for patients in each pathway regarding the following:

- Stroke
- Myocardial infarction
- Treatment complications
- Mortality

These are all objective measures. You might also be interested in measuring subjective aspects of care, which might include the patient's satisfaction with care, and aspects of quality of life and functional status.

Patients to be included in your outcomes study should represent all patients managed by the hospital physicians, not just those seen in the emergency room or admitted to the hospital, and not just those treated by neurologists.

4. Have them recognize that their strong opinions would best be heard at the time of the guideline development, so that they could have input into the ultimate drafting of them.

Also explain that guidelines can be helpful tools for protecting physicians facing potentially risky outcomes of care. If a clinician follows an accepted guideline and an adverse event occurs, he or she can cite the guideline in the case of a malpractice claim. In addition, try to gain his or her understanding of the necessity of cost control for the survival of the hospital, and suggest that his or her input is important to assure that cost control does not come at the expense of patient care. If all else fails, mandate participation on guidelines teams as a requirement for staff privileges.

Developing the Guideline

1. It is essential to involve all the clinicians involved in managing these patients, especially those from internal medicine and the emergency room. You need to find a time at which all can meet—perhaps you should reschedule your staff meeting time!

When clinicians admit rare patients with transient ischemic attack, it is more difficult to influence patient care with guidelines—the nursing staff on other floors might not be aware of the clinical pathways, and the physicians might be unaware of the guidelines or might not have been targeted for education and decision supports.

Implementing the Guideline

1. Endorsement by the key department chairs is necessary, but not sufficient, to ensure that the guideline can be operationalized. Further review by people in the "trenches"—those who are actually involved in the day-to-day operations of their departments—is necessary to ensure that availability of tests, turnaround times, scheduling conflicts, formulary compatibility, etc., do not disable the guideline. When system support problems are identified, they must be addressed by modifying either the guideline or the system before the guideline can be disseminated and implemented. This operational analysis can be accomplished by several methods that are best combined to ensure reliability.

Three major methods are operational analysis, failure mode effects analysis, and force field analysis. Operational analysis is a three-step process:

1. Review of the guidelines by the affected managers responsible for daily operations in their areas.
2. Review charts of patients with the clinical condition in question prior to the guideline implementation in order to see where their management would have differed had the guideline been applied. You should anticipate the volume of patients whose management will lead to different patterns of testing, nursing, etc.
3. Pilot the guideline in a small area, to note its changes on support resources, prior to widespread implementation.

2. See answer for part 3.2 in table A-7. The recognition of potential failures is more important than the actual assignment of numbers to the parameters, which is quite subjective. Nonetheless, recognizing limitations in reliability, the failure mode effects analysis ranking does tend to highlight major potential pitfalls that might otherwise be missed with a less exhaustive process.

The actual assignment of scores to each item, however, is best accomplished in a group setting to foster internal comparability. At the end of the prioritization, the group should go over the ordered list to check it for face validity. When making a quantitative rank ordering out of qualitative data, the list is only as good as the assumptions you put into it!

3. Doing a force field analysis is another way to compel yourself to examine potential implementation issues in a systematic and rigorous way. Recognition of the forces impacting clinician behavior, both positively and negatively, will allow you to design implementation supports that will enhance facilitating features and overcome restraints. Note possible implementation issues on the partially completed diagram in figure A-13.

4. Following are several support strategies:

- Suggest that leaders hold sessions with clinician staff on transient ischemic attack management.
- Develop a quiz related to the guideline that can be submitted for continuing medical education credits; require that all patients admitted for transient ischemic attack receive neurological consultation.
- Develop academic detailing, one-on-one, to emphasize the evidence that anticoagulation is not indicated for most patients.
- Target specific educational interventions for emergency room physicians, who determine patient dispositions, about indications for admissions.
- Consider economic incentives for clinicians to manage transient ischemic attack patients as outpatients.
- Develop educational materials for patients about transient ischemic attack.

TABLE A-7. Partially Completed Failure Mode Effects Analysis, II

Process Step	Potential Failure Mode	Possible Causes	Likelihood (L) (1–5)	Severity (S) (1–5)	Priority (L x S) (1–25)	Overall Effect
2. TIA (5d) or recurrent	Don't identify new TIA patient	Doctor not aware important	1.	3	3	High recurrence TIA or stroke
		Patient denies	1		3	High recurrence TIA or stroke
	Don't identify recurrent TIA patient	Doctor not aware important	2	4	8	High recurrence TIA or stroke
		Patient denies	1		4	High recurrence TIA or stroke
3.1 Expedited outpatient workup	Workup takes too long	Tests unavailable	4	3	12	High recurrence TIA or stroke
		Not ordered appropriately	2		6	High recurrence TIA or stroke
	Workup takes too long	Patient didn't keep appointment	1		3	High recurrence TIA or stroke
3.2 Indications for hospitalization	Not knowing indications	Did not receive guidelines	1	4	4	Inappropriate failure to hospitalize
		Did not learn guidelines	3		12	Inappropriate failure to hospitalize
	Failure to recognize indications	Did not take proper history	2	4	8	Same as above; possible worse outcome
		Does not know factors determining probable cardiac embolism	2		8	Same as above; possible worse outcome

FIGURE A-13. Force Field Diagram—Partially Completed

Driving Forces

Patient influences

Restraining Forces

Patient influences

Patient expectation for hospital

Patient distrust of healthy maturity

Personal influences

Personal influences

Desire good will of Chief

Fear of litigation

ER doctors want to clear beds, admit patients faster

Educational influences

Educational influences

Literature supports guideline

Traditional training

Economic influences

Economic influences

Imperative for hospital to save dollars

Decreased compensation for neurologist

Administrative influences

Administrative influences

Aggressive UR nurses

Limited access to off-hours CT, ultrasound

No site for urgent outpatient workup—

ER resists holding

Multiple specialties admitting

- Provide feedback to clinicians about patients seen for transient ischemic attack, correlating management and outcomes.
- Develop a "holding unit" for patients to be housed from the emergency room while undergoing workup.
- Attach guidelines to order form for computed tomography scan.
- Develop an on-call system for technicians and radiologists to be available during off-hours for workup.

Developing a Clinical Care Path

1. Team participants should include the following:

- Floor nurses
- Discharge planning nurses/social service
- Lab/radiology staff
- Neurology/internal medicine/surgery/cardiology medical doctors

The composition of the pathway team is different from that of a guidelines team because the clinical care pathway specifies details of routine care, provided by all hospital personnel who interact with management of the patient, rather than clinical decision making.

2. The path differs from the algorithm for the following reasons:

- There is little branching logic.
- Its emphasis is on timeliness rather than on clinical decision making.

It is similar to the algorithm for the following reasons:

- It specifies care for one arm of the clinical algorithm (hospitalized patients).
- It is unambiguous.
- It is a flow scheme, but presented as a table.
- It contains simple conditional logic such as, "If it is day one of the care process, then do . . . If it is day two, then do. . . ." Even within the routine steps, there is conditional logic—for example, "If it is day one within 12 hours of admission, consider initiating heparin."

It is necessary to have a guideline in designing a clinical care pathway—the guideline can be written out or (less rigorously) implicitly assumed. The guideline is essential to identifying which patients should enter the clinical path and how to determine the "if needed" components of the clinical path.

Elements essential to a clinical path that are not present in the process flow or guideline are as follows:

- Timing for interventions
- Identification of personnel involved in care
- Nursing orders

3. Because the clinical pathway addresses interventions within a confined setting (the hospital), its implementation is perhaps more straightforward than the guideline. An implementation recommendation might include the following instructions:

- Educate the caregivers specified by the pathway about its recommendations.
- Attach a copy of the pathway to each transient ischemic attack patient chart.
- Assign responsibility to a primary nurse to oversee the pathway, and remind clinicians when recommendations have not been implemented; develop a set of "standing orders" for patients with transient ischemic attack.
- Require a daily check-off of the protocol, and require a statement of variance when the clinical path is not followed.

Interpreting Data, Revising the Pathway, Spin-off Projects

1. The pre and post bar graphs show that most, but not all, neurologists have changed their admitting practices for transient ischemic attack patients. One might want to feed this information back to their neurologists. Neurologist D might be targeted for academic detailing, although it is possible that there is something about her patient base that justifies her relatively higher admission rate (perhaps she specializes in managing patients with cardiac disease). The histogram shows that the distribution is significantly narrowed, as well as shifted to the left, and there is now a normal distribution, which suggests a single process is in place.

2. The main issue here is case mix: one can't compare admitted and ambulatory patients for clinical outcomes without controlling for comorbidity, since there is certainly a selection process favoring healthier patients as nonadmits.

One might hypothesize the following about hospitalized patients:

- They have more heart disease
- They are older
- They are more likely to be anticoagulated
- They might have had a more significant neuro event
- They might be exposed to more iatrogenic events

One would want data on comorbidities, age distribution, and whether or not shorter stays correlated with adverse events.

The Coumadin data do not suggest that anticoagulation contributes significantly to the adverse event rate. While 15/52 (29 percent) patients taking Coumadin had an adverse event and 4/23 (17 percent) patients not taking Coumadin had an adverse event, given the small sample size the numbers are not significant.

The data are not sufficient to determine whether or not the guideline or pathway needs to be revised. It is not appropriate to compare adverse event rates for hospitalized patients before and after the guideline, because the guideline led to a sicker population being hospitalized, and there is no way to determine outcomes for patients who were not hospitalized before the database was developed. Certainly, one should continue to track clinical outcomes and the possible need for revision should be kept in mind.

3. A clinician group would need to determine whether or not there are justifiable reasons to delay introducing Coumadin to patients who are to be anticoagulated. If not, the pathway should be revised to move Coumadin to day one.

Note that both of the spin-off problems involve technical rather than clinical failure modes. Despite correct clinical decisions to use Heparin or Coumadin, anticoagulation is taking too long! The actual heparinization protocol chart developed is shown in exhibit A-1. Of course, clinical improvement involves both clinical and technical administrative modes.

EXHIBIT A-1. Heparinization Protocol Chart

PHYSICIANS ORDER SHEET	
DIAGNOSIS:	
PRIMARY:	
SECONDARY:	
DRUG ALLERGIES:	
☐ IN ACCORDANCE WITH OUR FORMULARY SYSTEM THE USE OF GENERIC EQUIVALENTS IS ACCEPTABLE UNLESS BOX IS CHECKED.	☐ SURGICAL ☐ ENT. ☐ NEURO ☐ OB-GYN ☐ MEDICAL ☐ OPHTHAL. ☐ DERMATOLOGY ☐ ORTHOPEDIC ☐ PEDIATRIC ☐ UROLOGY ☐ PSYCHIATRIC ☐ DENTAL ☐ OTHER (specify)
ORDERED: DATE: HOUR:	

HEPARIN ORDER SHEET
(All blanks must be filled in by physician)

1. Make calculations using total body weight: _____ kg.

2. BOLUS HEPARIN, 80 units/kg = _____ units IV.

3. IV HEPARIN infusion, 18 units/kg/hr = _____ units/hr.
   (25,000 units heparin in 500 ml of DSW = 50 units/ml)

4. LABORATORY: PTT, PT, CBC now
                       CBC with platelet count Q3 days
                       <u>STAT</u> PTT 6 hours after heparin bolus
                       PT Q day (start on third day of heparin)

5. Guaiac all stools.

6. ADJUST heparin infusion based on sliding scale below.

PTT <40	80 units/kg bolus = _____ units Increase drip 4 units/kg/hr = _____ units/hr
PTT 40–49	40 units/kg bolus = _____ units Increase drip 2 units/kg/hr = _____ units/hr
PTT 50–80	No change
PTT 81–100	Reduce drip 1 unit/kg/hr = _____ units/hr
PTT 101–120	Reduce drip 2 units/kg/hr = _____ units/hr
PTT 121–140	Hold heparin for 30 minutes Reduce drip 3 units/kg/hr = _____ units/hr
PTT >141	Hold heparin for 60 minutes Reduce drip 4 units/kg/hr = _____ units/hr

7. Order a PTT 6 hours after any dosage change, adjust heparin infusion by the sliding scale unit so PTT is within therapeutic range (50–80 sec.). When 2 consecutive PTTs are therapeutic, order PTT QD and adjust heparin accordingly.

<u>Please make changes as promptly as possible</u> and round off doses to the nearest ml/hr (nearest 50 units per hour).

SIGNATURE _____

Answers to Chapter Questions, and Solutions to Chapter Problems and Exercises

ANSWERS TO CHAPTER 1 QUESTIONS

1. A clinical algorithm is a step-by-step approach to solving a clinical problem.

2. The differences between mathematical and practical algorithms are illustrated below:

Characteristics of Algorithms

	Practical	Mathematical
Addresses all possible problem situations	–	+
Fuzzy language	+	–
Imprecise outcomes	+	–
Finite input	–	+

3. All the information relevant to a diagnostic and therapeutic approach to solving and caring for a patients' clinical problem.

4. A clinical algorithm is the logic engine of a clinical practice guide-line.

5. A job performance aid is a type of algorithm that provides pictures of key decision situations (for example, Tuddenham's algorithm).

6. A flowchart is one possible graphic format of algorithm presentation.

7. (1) Prose—graphic format/Used frequently in textbooks/An ineffective way to describe complex algorithms; (2) A list—graphic format/ Used to embed algorithm instructions into an encounter form;

(3) Verbal description/Frequently used at the bedside to describe or imply an algorithmic approach to a patient's problem.

8. To elucidate the approach to solving a clinical problem/To teach the approach/To guide clinicians while taking care of patients.

9. Only in the sense that they focus thinking on a specific approach to solving a specific problem. On the contrary, it may be argued that attempting to use such specific clinical problem solutions is essential to proper clinical decision making and may increase the clinician's ability to recognize an unusual problem.

10. (1) Clarity; (2) Usability; (3) Improvement of care and/or health (validity).

ANSWERS TO CHAPTER 2 QUESTIONS

1. When there is no general agreement about the approach to solving a clinical problem.

2. (1) Improving quality by decreasing irrational variation; (2) Controlling cost; (3) Reminding practitioners how to approach an unfamiliar problem.

3. (1) Clinical experience; (2) Consensus of experts; (3) Evidence.

4. (1) Generating/choosing a seed clinical algorithm; (2) Marshaling the evidence; (3) Consensus processing; (4) Revising the seed; (5) Reiterating steps 3 and 4; (6) Appointing a clinical practice guideline tender.

5. (1) To draw an algorithm map (flowchart) of the guideline logic; (2) To use a systematic set of questions or checklist to rate the guideline quality. An example of such a checklist, currently in use in the United Kingdom, can be found in this book.

6. (1) Reading recent reviews/book chapters; (2) Systematically collecting all relevant research literature; (3) Grading evidence and recommendations using the U.S. Preventive Services Task Force (tables 3-2 and 3-3) approach (or some other accepted system).

7. Nominal group process and Delphi process.

8. No; they are frequently used in tandem, starting with nominal group process and, after two or more nominal group processes, ending with Delphi.

9. Subject expertise, user interest, and algorithm writing expertise. There should not be less than two editors to encourage discourse and probably not more than three editors to discourage pointless cycling in the discourse.

10. While revising the draft, the editors can include or exclude material according to their own judgment, even if their decision flies in the face of the consensus group opinion. However, their decisions must be approved by the group.

11. The tender is the person, usually a clinician, who worries about and cares for all aspects of guideline development, including construction, literature update, and guideline revision. This person may also choose the guideline and be involved in monitoring implementation.

12. In-house and institutional "sign-off."

13. No; it is the draft that is ready to be processed to produce an implementation plan—and don't you forget it!

SOLUTIONS TO CHAPTER 2 PROBLEMS AND EXERCISES

Exercise 1: How to Draw an Algorithm Map

Figure 1-3 in chapter 1 is one version of the traffic light algorithm first drawn by Dr. Alvin Feinstein in his landmark review of clinical algorithms (*Yale Journal of Biological Medicine* 47 (1974): 5–32). In 1973, when Dr. Feinstein drew these, annotations and appropriate bibliographical references were not yet a standard part of clinical algorithms. Today, his lack of explanation for the terms "cogent reason" and "make new decision as the situation changes" would have to be considered serious technical errors, as would the lack of references of any sort.

Exercise 2: How to Draw a Clinical Algorithm Map

One version can be seen in exercise 1 of chapter 4.

Exercise 3: Algorithmization

FIGURE 2-1. Protocol for Management of Coronary Heart Disease—Algorithm Map Format

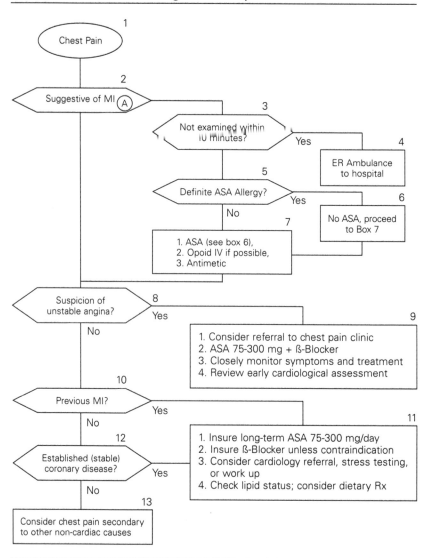

East Riding Health Authority Guideline (UK: May 1994).

Exercise 4: Algorithmization—Nonclinical

FIGURE 2-2. Leprosy Algorithm—Flowchart Format

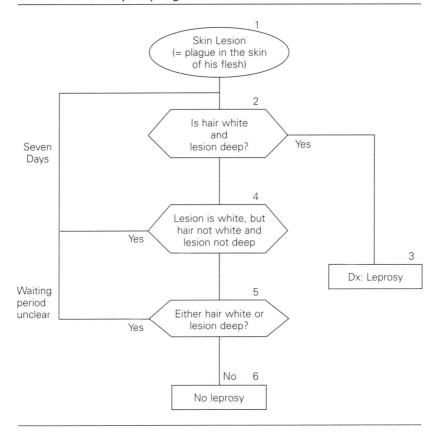

Exercise 5: Critiquing a Clinical Practice Guideline

Guideline appraisal: East Riding Health Authority
1. Y   2. N   3. NA   4. N   5. NA   6. N inadequate statement under
title 7. NA   8. N   9. NA   10. N   11. NA   12. N   13. N
14. NS   15. N   16. NS   17. N   18. N   19. Y   20. N   21. N
22. N   23. Y   24. N   25. N   26. Y   27. Y   28. Y   29. N
30. N   31. N   32. NA   33. N   34. N   35. Y   36. Y   37. N

ANSWERS TO CHAPTER 3 QUESTIONS

1. The composition of the guideline panel depends on the setting. In a care organization, the rule of thumb is that all major users should be represented. This might include subspecialty physicians, primary care physicians, nurses, nurse practitioners and physicians assistants, patients, and data analysts.

   In the setting of a national or state clinicians organization, such as specialty/organization or a state medical society, other experts that might be added are epidemiologists, behavior scientists, decision analysts, economists, and ethicists.

2. 1, How uncomfortable is the intervention? 2. How convenient is the intervention? 3. What are the risks? 4. What is the level of technical expertise available? 5. What are the costs of the intervention? 6. What is the cost-effectiveness of the intervention?

3. Unpublished work is less likely to report significant effects. Published work is biased toward positive findings.

4. Strong: randomized clinical trial; cohort study/Weak: case study; case series.

5. Measurement bias/Minimizing chance effects.

6. "Usual practice" has no place, but "mechanism of disease" can be helpful to understand the intervention.

7. Summarizing results of the best clinical studies/Systematic reviews (such as metanalysis)/Bradford-Hill criteria/Rating systems.

8. A major reason is that they have different values.

9. Scientific studies frequently deal with special populations, use "hard," measurable outcomes that may not be relevant, and tend not to report failures. Practitioners, on the other hand, may rarely see these populations and may be interested in "soft" outcomes, such as pain or nausea.

10. Proven effects include changing provider behavior, but the effect frequently is not of great magnitude. Unproven effects include the effect on cost. Although many studies have shown an effect on process, few have demonstrated an effect on outcome.

SOLUTIONS TO CHAPTER 4 PROBLEMS AND EXERCISES

Answers to Case 1

Pathway: 1 - 10 - 10a - 11 - 13 - 14

Outcome: Consider influenza; check immunization of debilitated patient (presumably not relevant in the patient).

Answers to Case 2

Pathway: 1 - 2 - 3

Outcome: Rule out peritonsillar abscess.

Answers to Case 3

Pathway: 1 - 2 - 3a - 3b

Outcome: Treat with penicillin, no culture. This woman with her acute pharyngitis and strong epidemiological evidence of streptococcal pharyngitis, should be treated. Culture is not necessary.

Answers to Case 4

Pathway: There is no pathway.

Outcome: Tony's problem is lower respiratory, not pharyngitis. Use another guideline or strategy.

Answers to Case 5

Pathway: 1 - 2 - 3a - 4 - 6 - 9

Outcome: Do throat culture, treat symptomatically.

Answers to Case 5a

Pathway: 1 - 2 - 3a - 4 - 6 - 7 - 12

Outcome: Do throat culture, begin penicillin, treat symptomatically.

Answers to Case 5b

Pathway: 1 - 2 - 3a - 4 - 6 - 7 - 8
Outcome: If penicillin started, stop it (continuation of case 5a).

Answers to Case 6

Pathway: 1 - 2 - 3a - 4 - 5
Outcome: Consider infectious mononucleosis.

Answers to Case 6a

Pathway: 1 - 2 - 3a - 4 - 5
Outcome: Consider cocksackie hand–foot–mouth infection.

ANSWERS TO CHAPTER 5 QUESTIONS

1. Local tailoring is critiquing and rewriting a template guideline so that it reflects line input and conditions at the clinical setting in which the guideline will be used.

2. Two purposes of tailoring: enable implementation and coopting implementors.

3. Three differences in the local setting that may require tailoring: a different prevalence of disease, a different care setting, local peculiarities of care (for example, local use of a specific antibiotic)

4. Nominal group process or Delphi.

5. No—the only exception would be if the evidence changed.

6. Any real clinical decision must be tailored to suit the patient. Local tailoring refers to changing a guideline decision, but when any guideline decision is made regarding a patient it will be tailored to that patient.

7. Local tailoring refers to tailoring one step down for a particular patient care setting. The guideline to be tailored may have been written for a global, national, or health maintenance organization audience. A

global one could be tailored at the national level, again at a health maintenance organization level, and even perhaps again at a clinic level within a health maintenance organization.

8. Both—it is the last guideline development step and the first step in implementation.

SOLUTIONS TO CHAPTER 5 PROBLEMS AND EXERCISES

Suggested Solution to Exercise 1

A possible strategy would involve the following steps:

1. Form a guideline team consisting of 7–10 players who are directly involved in diabetes care.

2. Do a nominal group process on the National Diabetes Association guideline.

3. Appoint a local guideline tender.

4. Have the tender and one or two other team members use the nominal group process comments to write the local version of the guideline.

5. Consider repeating the process or at least an abbreviated version of it at each clinic or group where the guideline will be used.

Solution to Exercise 2

The strategy would be similar to that in exercise 1. However, one would first check to determine whether a local organization guideline had already been developed. For example: Is the AIDS clinic part of a children's hospital; is there a hospital AIDS guideline? If there is, one would consider whether or not to further modify it. If no such local version exists, then one could proceed to do a nominal group process on the Agency for Health Care Policy and Research guideline in order to produce a local hospital guideline.

Guideline duplication has become a national malady. When the Agency for Health Care Policy and Research started to collect AIDS guidelines in preparation for making its own version, there were 56 versions available in 48 states. An obvious research question is, How many versions were duplicates?

Deciding which version of a guideline is the official template guideline would assist in diminishing duplication. The authors would be in favor of giving official status to guidelines developed by specialty societies and then upgrading the guideline capability of the societies.

INDEX

219